"One of the best books available for teaching patients how to cope with the challenges of cancer treatment. Everything, including how to understand diagnoses, treatment plans, and emotional and social challenges, is beautifully written in layman's terms so the patient can become an active partner in his or her own treatment. A must-read."

—Judith Shepherd, MSW, DSW, social worker at Alta Bates Summit Comprehensive Cancer Center

"The previous edition of this comprehensive, well-written guide was enthusiastically received by patients, nurses, and physicians. This updated edition is even more valuable. It contains information relating to all aspects of a potentially difficult and frightening diagnosis. The suggestions for symptom management are practical and constructive."

—Martha A. Tracy, MD, oncologist at Northern California Hematology Oncology Consultants

"This new edition of *The Chemotherapy Survival Guide* provides patients with practical ways to empower themselves, from beginning preparations for treatment to issues of survivorship. Its down-to-earth philosophy is an invaluable guide for health care providers who educate cancer patients."

—Quan Thai, RN, MSN, OCN, oncology nurse practitioner

"Besides being well organized and easy to read, *The Chemotherapy Survival Guide* has been a great comfort to me during my chemotherapy. It's the book I reach for when I get those late-night worries and questions."

—Susan Smith, cancer survivor

"*The Chemotherapy Survival Guide* should be read by all patients diagnosed with cancer as well as their families. It offers valuable information about cancer and the various approaches to therapy in addition to practical advice. This book will help readers understand the decisions they face, how to cope with the disease, and the treatments they will undergo."

—Michael Cassidy, MD, medical director at Alta Bates
Summit Medical Center Cancer Program

The Chemotherapy Survival Guide

THIRD EDITION

EVERYTHING YOU NEED TO KNOW TO GET THROUGH TREATMENT

JUDITH McKAY, RN, OCN
TAMERA SCHACHER, RN, OCN, MSN

New Harbinger Publications, Inc.

Publisher's Note

This publication is designed to provide accurate and authoritative information in regard to the subject matter covered. It is sold with the understanding that the publisher is not engaged in rendering psychological, financial, legal, or other professional services. If expert assistance or counseling is *needed, the services of a competent professional should be sought.*

Care has been taken to confirm the accuracy of the information presented and to describe generally accepted practices. However, the authors, editors, and publisher are not responsible for errors or omissions or for any consequences from application of the information in this book and make no warranty, express or implied, with respect to the contents of the publication.

The authors, editors, and publisher have exerted every effort to ensure that any drug selection and dosage set forth in this text are in accordance with current recommendations and practice at the time of publication. However, in view of ongoing research, changes in government regulations, and the constant flow of information relating to drug therapy and drug reactions, the reader is urged to check the package insert for each drug for any change in indications and dosage and for added warnings and precautions. This is particularly important when the recommended agent is a new or infrequently employed drug.

Some drugs and medical devices presented in this publication may have Food and Drug Administration (FDA) clearance for limited use in restricted research settings. It is the responsibility of the health care provider to ascertain the FDA status of each drug or device planned for use in their clinical practice.

Distributed in Canada by Raincoast Books

Copyright © 2009 by Judith McKay and Tamera Schacher
New Harbinger Publications, Inc.
5674 Shattuck Avenue
Oakland, CA 94609
www.newharbinger.com

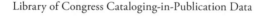

FSC
Mixed Sources
Product group from well-managed
forests and other controlled sources
Cert no. SW-COC-002283
www.fsc.org
© 1996 Forest Stewardship Council

All Rights Reserved
Printed in the United States of America

Acquired by Jess O'Brien; Cover design by Amy Shoup; Edited by Carole Honeychurch

Library of Congress Cataloging-in-Publication Data
McKay, Judith.
  The chemotherapy survival guide : everything you need to know to get through treatment / Judith McKay and Tamera Schacher. -- 3rd ed.
       p. cm.
Includes bibliographical references and index.
ISBN-13: 978-1-57224-621-8 (pbk. : alk. paper)
ISBN-10: 1-57224-621-9 (pbk. : alk. paper)
  1. Cancer--Chemotherapy--Popular works. I. Schacher, Tamera. II. Title.
RC271.C5M35 2009
616.99'4061--dc22

                      2008052321

11   10   09
10   9   8   7   6   5   4   3   2   1   First printing

For my daughter, Dana.

—J.Mc.

To the memory of my grandmother, Alvena Jenny, and my friend,
Therese Schoofs.

—T.S.

Contents

Acknowledgments

We are grateful to the following people, who have been extremely helpful in developing this book: Michael Cassidy, MD; Cheryll Willin, MSN, AOCN; Eun Jeong Kim, Pharm.D.; and Ann Katz, RN, Ph.D. They shared their expertise and gave us valuable feedback on several chapters.

We appreciate the contributions of Tinrin Chew, RD, CSO, and Burton A. Presberg, MD, whose chapters are included in this edition.

We would also like to thank all our patients and their families, who taught us so much. Their courage, struggles, and victories were our inspiration.

Introduction

A survival guide is a book of directions that helps people cope with difficulties or unusual circumstances. It provides essential information, practical suggestions, and encouragement so that they can use their own resources and those in their environments to make it through the obstacles along the way.

Many people who are facing cancer therapy for the first time feel as if they've been dropped off behind enemy lines during a war. They don't know the language or the terrain and don't know what to expect or what's expected of them. The hospital or clinic environment and the technical medical terminology are foreign. All these things add to the feeling of being lost in an alien world. A person recovering from the stress of recent cancer surgery may feel even more overwhelmed. And it may be difficult to get needed support if friends and family are dealing with their own fears and misconceptions about cancer and cancer-fighting treatments.

This book is meant to be a survival guide. It explains what chemotherapy is, how it works, and how it may affect you. It contains simple and understandable answers for many of the questions you may have. Most importantly, it gives you practical suggestions about what you can do to help yourself while receiving treatment. These are the same hints and suggestions that nurses give their patients based on their own experience and the experiences of the many people who've gone through these treatments.

CANCER-FIGHTING TREATMENTS

Before chemotherapy, the most common treatment for cancer was surgery. But if the cancer was in an area that couldn't be surgically removed, or if some cancer cells had spread to other areas of the body, no effective treatment was available. In those days, surgery tended to be more radical, often removing large areas of healthy tissue in an attempt to catch the few microscopic cancer cells that might have escaped from the original tumor.

One distinguishing characteristic of most cancer cells is their tendency to divide frequently—too frequently—in a way that's out of control. This tendency means that any drug or treatment that can damage cells in the dividing stage will have a far greater effect on cancer cells than on most normal tissue.

Chemotherapy is the term used to identify the various drugs that fight cancer. Some of these drugs travel throughout the body and can damage rapidly dividing cells (like cancer cells) so that tumors can't continue to grow. These drugs do that by interfering with the cell's life cycle at different stages. Many of the side effects of chemotherapy are caused by the chemotherapy's effect on normal cells that are also dividing frequently, such as the cells of the digestive tract or the bone marrow (where blood cells are produced). The first chemotherapy treatments used this principle to kill frequently dividing cells in the blood (leukemia) and the lymphatic system (lymphoma).

Since then, many more cancer-fighting drugs have been developed. Some can target a particular characteristic unique to the cancer so that normal cells are spared. Others stimulate your body's natural immunity to control or kill cancer cells. Researchers continue to explore how to use these and other drugs alone and in combination to make treatments even more effective.

Radiation therapy is the term used to identify the cancer-fighting treatment that uses high-energy rays (emitted by radioactive sources) to kill cancer cells. Radiation interacts with the atoms and molecules in the cell and either kills the cell or damages it so that it can't reproduce. Cells that divide frequently, such as tumor cells, are generally more sensitive to the effects of radiation. Radiation was first used to treat skin cancer, but today, high-energy radiation and modern methods can deliver treatment to tumors that lie deep within the body as well. Unlike chemotherapy, radiation does not affect cells throughout the body, only the ones in the area exposed to the radiation. Many of the side effects of radiation therapy are associated with its effect on normal tissue that may also be exposed to radiation during the treatments.

Modern chemotherapy and radiation therapy are powerful and, in many cases, highly effective weapons in the fight against cancer. For some kinds of cancer that are particularly vulnerable to the effects of radiation therapy, it may be the only treatment necessary. For other kinds of cancer, chemotherapy alone is sufficient to kill cancer cells, prevent the spread of the disease, and significantly improve the chances for recovery. Many people receive both chemotherapy and radiation therapy along with other forms of treatment, such as surgery and hormonal therapy. Sometimes chemotherapy or radiation therapy is recommended even when all measurable signs of cancer are gone. This is just to make sure that any possible spread of cancer cells—even on a microscopic level—is eliminated.

WHAT THIS BOOK OFFERS

Most people know very little about what to expect when they get chemotherapy. They may be aware of some potential side effects, such as nausea or hair loss, but they don't know what, if anything, they can do if these reactions occur.

The purpose of this book is to answer many of your questions about cancer and chemotherapy. Moreover, this book offers guidance for how to help yourself during your treatment. How is chemotherapy given? What should you do before, during, and after each treatment? What can you expect at home? Why do you need so many blood tests? What do the tests show about how your body is reacting to the treatments?

You don't need to read this book from beginning to end; you can turn to a particular chapter for information and suggestions about the specific issue that concerns you. It may be helpful for you, however, to read the first two or three chapters to familiarize yourself with the terminology used throughout this book.

Chapter 1 ("What Is Chemotherapy?") explains the basic facts about chemotherapy and how it works to kill cancer cells, the side effects that you can expect, and the reason these side effects may occur. Chapter 2 ("Understanding Your Treatment Plan") explains how a treatment plan is developed, the significance of diagnostic tests, and the questions to ask so that you understand the plan. Chapter 3 ("Understanding Blood Tests") explains the reasons for and significance of the many blood tests you may need during your treatment. Chemotherapy is often administered into a vein (a technique referred to as *intravenous* or *IV*). Chapter 4 ("The IV Experience") provides information about the different kinds of IVs and how they work, problems that may arise, and coping strategies to help you get through it all.

At the heart of this survival guide are chapters (5 and 6 and 8 through 12) describing the different side effects that might occur because of the way chemotherapy affects healthy cells. At the beginning of each of these chapters is an explanation of why the chemotherapy can cause that specific side effect, followed by many suggestions for how to prevent, minimize, or manage the side effect.

Chapter 7 ("Maintaining Good Nutrition"), written by Tinrin Chew, RD, CSO, an experienced oncology nutritionist, focuses on how to maintain good nutrition even when you're experiencing temporary changes in your appetite or digestion. Chapter 13 ("Mind and Body") was written by Burton A. Presberg, MD, a psychiatrist with many years of experience in counseling patients and families who are dealing with the stress of cancer treatments. Chapter 14 ("Relaxation and Stress Reduction") provides relaxation and stress-reduction techniques to lower your anxiety, and chapter 15 ("Preparing to Start Chemo: A Practical Guide") offers good suggestions to help you prepare for your first chemo treatment. Finally, chapter 16 ("Life After Cancer Treatments: Being a Survivor") addresses the important and sometimes surprising issues that arise after your treatment is over.

WHAT THIS BOOK CAN'T DO

This book doesn't include information about the individual chemo-therapy drugs or combinations of drugs used to treat specific kinds of cancer. Your doctor will prescribe the chemotherapy medications and dosages based on the kind of cancer you have, its location, and its cel-lular characteristics, as well as your age, your physical condition, and how well you're tolerating the treatment. Because so many different drugs, dosages, and combinations are now used to fight cancer, this book doesn't include descriptions of each drug. Your doctor or nurse will provide you with that information and review the potential side effects for each specific drug. If your treatment plan includes radiation therapy (before, during, or following chemo treatment), the radiation oncologist and the nurses will give you information about that phase of your treatment, which is beyond the scope of this book.

The Chemotherapy Survival Guide is not a substitute for calling the doctor if you have a problem. Many things about your treatment or symptoms may need the physician's immediate attention. What you may consider to be just a little cough or a cold may require antibiotics or lab tests when you're getting chemotherapy. An ache, a swelling, or a rash can also be more significant during cancer-fighting therapy. So don't be shy about calling with a problem, symptom, or question. Keep in mind that you'll probably develop a closer connection with your oncologist and the nurses in the oncology clinic than you may have had with health care providers in the past.

Cancer therapy is stressful, both physically and emotionally. But if you know what to expect, you'll feel less overwhelmed. If you understand what problems may arise and what you can do to feel better, you'll feel more empowered. If you're armed with practical suggestions and a coping plan to deal with problems, you can feel more in control. This survival guide can help make the journey easier by providing the information and sources of support you need to face the challenge and make it through.

Chapter 1

What Is Chemotherapy?

To understand how chemotherapy will help you, first you must understand how cancer cells differ from normal cells, how cancer cells grow, and how their growth can be stopped.

A PRIMER ON CELL LIFE

All living things are made up of cells, and each cell has a life of its own. Cells are the basic building blocks of life. When you look at a one-celled organism (like the amoeba you may have seen under the microscope in biology class), you can identify different cell structures that keep the cell working, dividing, and surviving. A cell wall surrounds the cell, separating it from its environment and determining what goes in and out. Within the cell is a very important structure called the *nucleus*, which is the cell's command center. The nucleus directs and controls all of a cell's functions, and determines how and when it divides. Within the nucleus is the *DNA*, which is like a master computer program for that cell.

When the cell divides, it splits into two identical pieces. First, the DNA splits in half and duplicates itself so that each half will have a complete and identical DNA program for that cell. Then the cell membrane and all the other structures divide. Each new "daughter" cell is exactly like the original "parent" cell, with identical cell parts, nucleus, and DNA information.

Complex life-forms like ourselves are made up of billions of cells. Groups of cells perform different specialized functions to keep the whole system working well. Some cells are part of the heart muscle and have the ability to contract. Other cells are part of the digestive system and secrete enzymes or absorb nutrients. Some are part of the liver and function to filter the blood and store energy. But all cells work together to keep the big system, the human body, alive and well in its environment. All cells are living, growing, and at times dividing in a specific and controlled way based on a program contained in the DNA.

Characteristics of Normal Cells

Normal cells grow in a limited space and stay within their boundaries. Bone cells don't grow into the muscles that surround them, and stomach cells don't grow into the space that the pancreas occupies (even though they lie right next to each other).

Normal cells divide at a set and controlled rate, depending on their function, their life span, and the information contained in their DNA. Some cells have a short life span and divide frequently. For example, the life span of some white blood cells is only seventy-two hours. The life span of a cell in your intestines is only two weeks. Other cells have a longer life span. The average red blood cell lives three to four months.

Some cells live as long as you do, dividing only to replace themselves if there has been an injury. For instance, if an adult breaks an arm, the bone cells are "turned on" to repair the damage. Once the injury heals, the bone cells go back to dividing only very rarely. In fact, there are some cells that never divide again once they've grown to adult size. Brain cells don't divide and replace themselves even when damaged. The rate at which normal cells divide is specific to each group and strictly controlled by its DNA program. This program is different for each type of cell.

Normal cells have a tendency to stick together so that cells don't break off and float away, even though the blood flows by each and every cell. If a normal cell were to break off into the blood and lodge elsewhere in the body, it would soon die. Normal cells are *well differentiated*, which means that for any normal cell, a pathologist (a lab doctor who examines body tissues and secretions) can easily identify what kind of cell it is, what it does, and where it comes from. Liver cells look different than bladder cells do; bone cells are quite distinct from brain cells. Cells with different functions vary in size, shape, and diameter of the nucleus.

How Cells Are Nourished

Every one of the body's cells is washed continuously with blood. The blood brings oxygen from the lungs and nutrients from the digestive system. The blood is pumped by the heart through big arteries, then smaller and smaller vessels, until the blood reaches each and every cell, delivering oxygen and energy. Then, the blood picks up waste products produced by the cells and carries them to the filtering and cleansing organs (kidneys, liver, and lungs) to be recycled or eliminated by the body. Every time you exhale, you get rid of some of the waste products (carbon dioxide) of cell activity. And when you urinate, you're eliminating waste products filtered out by your kidneys. Your blood is really a kind of transport system that trucks in life-sustaining supplies and then hauls off the debris.

How Cells Are Protected

Your immune system protects you by identifying and destroying foreign organisms and worn or damaged cells. It provides a mobile defense for the body, sending out white blood cells (you might call them "soldier cells") that seek and destroy bacteria and viruses. These cells are mixed in the blood and wash past every cell. They gather at sites of infection, surrounding and killing bacteria and viruses, and eventually migrate by way of lymph ducts to the lymph glands (or lymph nodes).

Lymph nodes occur in a cluster or chain and act as filtering stations at various locations in your body. Each cluster of nodes receives *lymphocytes* (one type of white blood cell) that have washed past a certain organ. The lymph nodes are the places where the bacteria, worn-out lymphocytes, and debris are filtered and destroyed. You aren't usually aware of your lymph nodes unless they're swollen and tender from fighting infection. For example, you might feel swollen lymph nodes in your neck or under your jaw from a sore throat or an infected tooth. You might feel lymph nodes in your groin from a pelvic infection or in your armpit from an infection in your hand. Doctors know where to find the particular cluster of lymph nodes that filter each organ. They know where to feel for signs of infection and which lymph nodes to examine under the microscope when looking for cancer cells.

Foreign cells (like bacteria and viruses) are identified by markings on their surface called *antigens*. The presence of the antigens stimulates your immune system to custom-make *antibodies* that will attach to the surface of the antigen and neutralize or destroy it. That is how vaccines work. They prevent you from developing a serious disease such as measles, mumps, or polio. The vaccine is an altered (weak or dead) form of the antigen that *does not cause the disease* but stimulates your body to develop antibodies against that antigen. These antibodies can stay in your system for years after you're vaccinated. Therefore, if you're ever exposed to the real disease-producing form of the antigens, you'll have the antibodies ready and able to destroy them before they can make you sick.

CHARACTERISTICS OF CANCER CELLS

Cancer begins as a mutation or change in the DNA of a group of normal cells in any part of the body. Once this change takes place, the set of instructions in the DNA is changed and the cell no longer acts like it normally does. Often a mutation or change results in a cell that's so damaged that it can't survive or it fails to divide successfully. But if it does survive and divide, that mutated cell (and any "daughter" cells) may look different and act very differently from the cells around it. It may have a different size or shape, or a larger or smaller nucleus.

It may not fit with other cells in an orderly, predictable arrangement. It may not be able to do the job that it was designed to do.

Even though a cancer cell is not a "foreign" cell, like a bacterium or virus, and is not usually targeted by your immune system, some tumor cells have abnormal surfaces that act like antigens.

Cancer cells often ignore the normal rate of cell division, because they lack a growth-control mechanism. They may divide very rapidly, crowding, pushing, or blocking other organs and preventing them from doing their jobs. Because they don't stay within their boundaries, but instead grow into surrounding organs, they're said to be *invasive*. Cancer cells frequently appear immature, because they may divide several times before they're fully grown. They're also more likely to mutate again.

Whereas normal cells have a tendency to stick together, cancer cells are more likely to detach from the original location and move, via the bloodstream, to other areas of the body. They're also more likely to travel by way of the lymphatic system to the lymph nodes downstream and then to other organ systems. Usually, many of these detached cells are destroyed by the body's defense system, or filtered and eliminated like bacteria and other cell debris. But if the detached cancer cells do survive, they may produce a new growth at a different site or damage other organs as well.

Some Common Terms

Here's a brief introduction to some terms used to describe cell growth.

Hyperplasia is an increase in the number of cells at a particular site. It's a normal healing response to an injury, such as a broken bone or a surgical incision. It means that the cells grow and divide more quickly until the bone or incision is healed, when growth can slow down to its usual pace. The cells grow in an orderly, regular way and are easily identifiable (well differentiated). They look and act like normal cells.

Dysplasia is an overgrowth of cells that don't have the arrangement or function of normal cells. *Neoplasia* means new growth and describes the growth of cells beyond their normal boundaries. These new cells may be cancerous (*malignant*) or noncancerous (*benign*). Noncancerous overgrowths of cells are well differentiated, and the cells look similar to other normal cells of the same organ. Such a growth usually divides slowly and is often encased in a limited area. It doesn't invade the tissue around it, nor will it travel to any other parts of the body. A benign cyst is an example of a noncancerous neoplasia.

A *malignant tumor* is an overgrowth of cells that often looks very dissimilar to normal cells in that organ. The cells may appear immature, divide quickly, and grow in a less orderly way. They may not be enclosed in a limited area and can invade the surrounding tissue. They can also detach from the tumor into the lymphatic or circulatory system and migrate to distant parts of the body. Some may survive and begin dividing in this new region.

Cancerous cells that have detached and traveled by the circulatory or lymphatic system often can't survive the body's defense systems. Occasionally, however, they may lodge in an area where the blood pressure is low and blood moves slowly. Then the cancerous cells may grow there. This spread of cancer cells to a distant organ site is called *metastasis*.

DIAGNOSIS

From the very beginning, a doctor wants to know everything possible about the cancer to determine the most effective treatment plan. You'll probably go through a number of diagnostic tests before your treatment begins.

Biopsy

When a little bit of a tumor is removed and examined under a microscope, this procedure is called a *biopsy*. A pathologist looks at a few cells from the tumor to see how they compare to normal cells of that organ, and to determine whether the tumor has invaded surrounding tissue. By looking at nearby lymph nodes, the patholo-gist can see if parts of the tumor have detached and are growing there. Even the DNA of the cancer cell is examined to help precisely diagnose the type of cancer based on the genes and proteins involved in the abnormal cell growth.

Staging

Your doctor may also order other tests, such as X-rays, scans, and blood tests. This information-gathering process is called *staging*. These tests give your doctor information about how well your body's other systems are working, as well as indicate any other places where cancer cells may be growing.

TREATMENT CHOICES

Once your doctor has all the diagnostic information, a treatment plan can be developed.

Surgery

This is the oldest method of treating cancer, and sometimes it's the only treatment necessary. This is more likely to be true if the cancer is small, is contained, and hasn't spread to adjacent tissue or through the lymphatic or circulatory system to a distant site. At the time of surgery, the tumor is removed along with some of the healthy surrounding tissue. Often lymph nodes from adjacent areas are also removed so that the pathologist can see if they have some cancerous cells growing in them.

If the cancer has spread, or if it's an aggressive type of cancer with a high likelihood of spreading to other organs, additional anticancer treatments may be recommended. In many cases, these additional treatments are recommended even if the original cancer is small, is contained, and shows no sign of spreading to other areas.

Radiation

This treatment uses high-energy particles that can penetrate body tissues. Special machines generate and direct these particles to a specific place for a specific amount of time. A specialist (the *radiation oncologist*) calculates the exact area, amount, and frequency of radiation treatments based on the kind of tumor and its location. Normal tissues are shielded, and the radiation beam is precisely aimed at the tumor so that it gets a high dose of radiation and the normal tissue does not. Radiation damages the cell's DNA, cell membranes, and other cell structures. Cells that divide frequently, like cancer cells, are especially sensitive to radiation. When high-energy particles are directed at a tumor, they damage or destroy these cells.

Radiation may be the only treatment necessary if the cancer cells are very sensitive to its effects and there's no sign that the cancer has spread.

Radiation treatment may be given *before* surgery to shrink a tumor so that it can more easily be removed. Or, it may be given *along with* or *following* chemotherapy. Some of the chemotherapy medicines make cancer cells more sensitive to the effects of radiation. Radiation may be suggested after surgery even if there are no detectable cancer cells in the lymph or surrounding tissue, just to make sure no cells have escaped.

Chemotherapy

The medicines used to treat cancer include a large number of different drugs. Some, like steroids, have familiar uses other than the treatment of cancer. But any drug or combination of drugs that kills, slows down, or damages cancer cells can be considered chemotherapy.

You're familiar with medicines that treat bacterial infection, such as antibiotics. Once they enter your bloodstream, these drugs usually have little effect on the rest of your body. It's the bacteria that are sensitive to and killed by the antibiotics. But since cancer cells are not foreign invaders, but instead are damaged, mutated human cells, anticancer medicine has to work in a different way. It has to kill cancer cells without permanently damaging normal cells.

Some chemotherapy drugs interfere with the sequence of activities that a cell must go through to divide into two identical daughter cells. If the cell can't divide, then it will live out its life span and die. Drugs that act this way are called *cell-cycle specific*. They prevent cancer cells from reproducing at a particular phase of the cell's life span.

Other chemotherapy drugs affect cancer cells in all phases of life. But because cancer cells are often more immature or fragile than normal cells, these drugs affect cancer cells far more than healthy cells. These medicines are called *cell-cycle nonspecific* since they kill cancer cells at any time during the cell's life span without waiting for them to divide.

Other drugs can make the environment less hospitable to cancer cells and thus slow them down. Hormone-blocking medicines work this way. For instance, some breast cancer tumors grow faster in the presence of estrogen, and some prostate cancers grow faster in the presence of testosterone. Hormones that block estrogen or testosterone can discourage the growth of those cancer cells.

Targeted Therapies

As just described, many chemotherapy medicines work by damaging cells that divide frequently. But other normal cells in the body also divide frequently. Even though cancer cells are generally more sensitive to the effects of chemotherapy and radiation, researchers are always looking for some way to *target* cancer cells specifically while leaving normal cells alone. And they're looking for ways to stimulate your natural immune system to fight cancer.

Some targeted therapies focus on blocking the signals that tell cancer cells to grow and divide uncontrollably, or they attempt to interfere with the molecules that cause normal cells to become cancer cells.

Monoclonal antibodies and anticancer vaccines stimulate your normal immune system (white cells, antibodies, and so on) to identify and attack cancerous cells.

Interferons are natural proteins produced in your body in response to viruses, bacteria, and tumors. Manufactured forms of interferon given in high doses work by inhibiting cell growth, strengthening the body's immune system, and reducing the cancer cells' resistance to the immune system.

As a tumor grows, it needs to develop a larger blood supply. *Anti-angiogenesis* drugs slow down the growth of the tumor by keeping it from developing new blood vessels.

Some drugs enhance your body's ability to recover from the effects of chemotherapy by stimulating the repair and recovery of healthy cells.

Targeted therapy can be used alone or in combination with chemotherapy to make treatment more effective.

Combinations of Drugs

Years ago, people were usually given one chemotherapy drug at a time. Now, with further research and the development of new drugs and therapies, doctors may recommend a combination of chemotherapy treatments. Using a combination of drugs can often be more effective at killing cancer cells than using one drug alone. Anticancer drugs with different modes of action and those that produce different side effects are usually combined. For instance, you may be given a chemotherapy drug that kills the cancer cells as they divide, and you may also be given a chemotherapy drug that kills cells even when they're not dividing. You may also take a hormone-blocking agent, which will change the environment of the cancer cells and discourage their growth. Your treatment plan might include a monoclonal antibody or another targeted therapy as well.

Using a combination of drugs that work in different ways can make chemotherapy more deadly to cancer cells and less toxic to healthy cells. The specific drug or combination of drugs recommended, as well as the schedule of how frequently you get treatments, depends on a number of things: the kind of cancer, the particular medication you're given, and how quickly your healthy cells recover from the treatment.

SIDE EFFECTS OF CHEMOTHERAPY

You take medicine for some desired effect. Different medicines can lower blood pressure, relieve pain, kill bacteria, and so on. The effects are usually predictable and beneficial. But medicines often have other effects, which may be predictable but aren't necessarily beneficial. Side effects are undesired consequences that may occur when taking certain medicines.

For instance, while the predictable and beneficial effect of a narcotic is to relieve pain, one of its side effects is sleepiness. You're often informed of the side effects of common medications when they're prescribed.

Since many chemotherapy medicines work by damaging cells that divide frequently, we can predict that these medicines will have an effect on the normal, noncancerous cells in your body that also divide frequently. These are cells of the bone marrow (where blood cells are made) and the mucous membranes of the gastrointestinal (GI) tract (from the mouth to the large intestine). Hair follicle cells also divide frequently, and they're sensitive to some chemotherapy medicines. The side effects of these kinds of chemotherapy medicines reflect the effect they have on all fast-growing cell populations.

Most chemotherapy medicines temporarily affect the ability of the bone marrow to produce blood cells, including the white blood cells that fight infection. Some chemotherapy medicines temporarily cause digestive disturbances such as diarrhea, nausea, or vomiting. Some chemotherapy medicines cause temporary hair loss or hair thinning, as well as changes in skin and nails. Chemotherapy medicines that stimulate your immune system can cause a fever or achy flu-like symptoms.

The kind of side effects you may experience depends on the kind of chemotherapy drugs you're getting, the dose, and the frequency of your treatments. Your doctor and nurse will tell you what you can expect with each recommended drug or treatment. It's most important to remember that most of the side effects of chemo are temporary.

IN CONCLUSION

Because chemotherapy goes all through your body, it can destroy cancer cells wherever they may be hiding. Side effects are the result of chemo's effect on other, normal cells in your body. Some side effects are *preventable*. For instance, the side effect of nausea can often be prevented by taking antinausea medication before getting chemo, and for several doses afterward. Some side effects can't be prevented, but there are still many things that you can do to minimize, relieve, or manage them.

Preventing and managing the side effects of chemotherapy is important. When you can eat, drink, and sleep well, your healthy cells recover more quickly. Knowing what to expect and how to prevent and manage the side effects of treatment will make things less overwhelming and help your spirits as well.

Chapters 5 to 6 and 8 to 12 will tell you much more about the possible side effects of chemotherapy. They explain why the side effects occur and what you can do to manage problems if they occur.

Chapter 2

Understanding Your Treatment Plan

In preparing for any battle, you want to know as much about the enemy as you can. You want to know its location, resources, habits, and weaknesses. From that information, you can develop a plan of attack that will give you the best chance of success.

FOUNDATIONS OF THE TREATMENT PLAN

Your treatment plan is your doctor's recommendation of the best way to kill cancer cells and, if possible, prevent their recurrence. The plan will depend on information about the cancer cells (information from the pathology report) and whether or not cancer may be affecting other parts of your body (results of scans and blood tests).

Factors such as your age, sex, health, and family history are very important. Your doctor will want to know about any other medical problems you dealt with before you had cancer: problems such as diabetes, heart disease, high blood pressure, kidney trouble, allergies, skin conditions, digestion issues—everything. Do you have pain, numbness, or difficulty breathing? Are you eating normally? Are you still recovering from surgery? What medicines are you taking? Your doctor will ask you questions about your "lifestyle." Do you drink or smoke, and how often? Are you active? Are you working? Have other people in your family had cancer? Your first visit to the oncologist will include a thorough interview and physical exam. As mentioned, this process of information gathering is called "staging," and the results of all these tests guide your doctor in developing your treatment plan.

The Pathology Report

When you were first diagnosed, you probably had surgery to remove all or part of the cancer. Samples may have been taken from areas around the tumor, including lymph nodes, to determine if the cancer had spread to adjoining areas. If your cancer arose from the blood- or lymph-producing places in your body, you may have had a biopsy of your bone marrow, where the various blood cells are produced.

Specialists known as *pathologists* work in the lab and examine tumor cells visually and microscopically. They report on the size of the tumor, what organ it came from, and how similar or different it is compared to normal cells. They can tell if it's invasive (likely to spread) and its rate of growth. They also may test the cancer cells for changes in DNA or the presence of hormone receptors. The pathologist's report includes similar information about any lymph nodes that were removed during surgery or biopsy.

Scans and X-Rays

Your doctor may send you for scans to check for abnormalities in other areas of your body. Cells from the original tumor may have traveled through your bloodstream or lymphatic system to another place (liver, lungs, bones, and so on). Sometimes these scans reveal abnormalities that have *nothing to do* with cancer. They may show cysts, old fractures, or arthritis. Specialists known as *radiologists* know how to "read" (interpret) the images and give an assessment. Whether or not abnormalities are found, results of diagnostic scans are important as baseline information in determining your treatment plan. Later, future scans can be compared to them. Here are some ways the doctor can evaluate the inside of your body from the outside:

- *X-rays* give a two-dimensional image of the inside of your body—your bones, teeth, lungs, and other organs.

- *Computed tomography* (or *CT*) scans give a three-dimensional image of the inside of your body from a series of X-rays around a single axis.

- *Positron emission tomography* (or *PET*) scans use a radioactive material to measure body functions such as glucose (sugar) metabolism to show how well organs and tissues are functioning.

- *Magnetic resonance imaging* (or *MRI*) scans use a magnetic field to provide an image that can show the contrast between different soft tissues, including the brain, muscles, bones, and blood vessels.

- *Bone scans* use a radioactive material to visualize abnormalities in bones. These scans can detect the presence of tumor, fracture, or infection.

- *Ultrasound* (or *sonography*) uses sound waves to visualize internal organs, muscles, and bone surfaces, as well as to delineate fluid-filled spaces in the body.

Lab Tests

A sample of your blood (or other body fluids) analyzed in the lab provides important information when developing a treatment plan. For instance, it can indicate how well your bone marrow is producing blood cells. Or, it can indicate the presence of infection as well as the health of your vital organs. *Tumor markers* are substances in your blood that are sometimes associated with certain kinds of cancer. Analysis of urine, stool, sputum, or wound drainage can give the doctor information about infection or abnormal bleeding. Chapter 3 ("Understanding Blood Tests") has more information about the importance of lab tests and what they indicate about your health.

Treatment Conference

Some hospitals or regional cancer centers have a forum where different kinds of cancer specialists meet to discuss a patient's treatment plan. This may be called a *treatment conference* or *tumor board*. The group of experts may include medical oncologists, radiation oncologists, pathologists, surgeons, and cancer researchers. After discussing your case, they may issue a report covering all the recommendations for treatment and follow-up care. Some hospitals refer all their new patients for this review. Or you may ask your oncologist if it's available in your area and whether this would be useful for you.

DECIDING ON THE TREATMENT PLAN

During your next visit, your doctor may recommend chemotherapy alone or in combination with radiation therapy, hormonal therapy, targeted therapy, or surgery. Your doctor will explain treatment options and why a certain one is recommended. Your doctor may be able to show you statistics (gathered over many years from all over the world) that indicate the advantage of one treatment over other available treatments, or the risk (if any) of not getting treatment.

Questions to Ask About Your Treatment Plan

Once all the relevant information is gathered and reviewed, you'll probably have another appointment with your doctor and another chance to ask questions. Many people feel better prepared to ask questions at this interview than when they first met their oncologists. For instance, you'll have had more time to learn about the kind of cancer you're dealing with, the treatment options available, many of the relevant medical terms and abbreviations used, and the significance of tests. You may also have had the opportunity to talk to other people who've gone through a similar treatment. When other questions occur to you, write them down so that you don't forget to ask about the things that concern you.

Here are some questions you may want to ask your doctor:

- What's the expected goal of the treatment? Is it to eliminate all cancer cells and prevent their recurrence? Is the goal to slow down the spread of cancer that can't be totally eliminated in order to achieve a remission (period of time when the cancer is inactive) for as long as possible? Is the goal to relieve the symptoms associated with the cancer (pain, shortness of breath, problems with digestion, and so on)?

- Do I need other kinds of treatments (surgery, radiation therapy, targeted therapy, hormonal treatment, and so on)? Why?

- What are the names of the chemotherapy medications I'll get?

- How many treatments will I be getting? How often will they be given? How long does each treatment take?

- What side effects can I expect (hair loss, nausea, increased risk of infection, or fatigue)? How can these side effects be prevented? How can they be managed?

- How will the treatment affect my other medical conditions (diabetes, heart disease, lung problems, kidney problems, and so on)?

- How will this treatment affect my sexuality? Fertility? Will these effects be temporary or permanent?

- Will I be able to continue to work? Travel?

- How will I know if the treatment plan is working? What tests will I need and how often?

Getting Your Questions Answered

When you're first diagnosed, you may not even know what questions to ask. And the answer to one question often leads to many more questions about things you may not have considered before.

It's hard to take in a lot of new information when you feel anxious. It's normal to need information to be clarified and repeated often during this time. Don't hesitate to say, "You may have answered this before, but I need you to tell me again about _____."

You may find that while the doctor is addressing one important concern, you forget to ask about another. Here are a few suggestions to help you avoid confusion and get the most out of your consultation:

Bring a list of your questions. Write down your questions as they occur to you. You might forget them over time, especially if there are several weeks between your doctor's appointments. Before your appointment, organize the questions into categories so that you can ask about one subject at a time. You may find that the answer to one question answers the other questions in that category.

Jot down new information. Write down just the essentials in an abbreviated way. Don't try to write everything down, because then you'll be too busy to fully hear or relate to the answers. You may need to write down the name of a consulting doctor (such as a surgeon or radiologist), the names of medications, the number of treatments recommended, how to reach the nutritionist, and so on. Some people bring a tape recorder to visits where they'll be discussing treatment decisions or getting a lot of new information. You can ask if it's okay to record the session.

Repeat what you heard to be sure that you understand. You can eliminate so much confusion (and worry) if you clarify what you've heard. You may need some things repeated or redefined so that they're clear to you. Then repeat them again in your own words.

Report all your symptoms (even if you think some of them aren't directly related to your treatments). Let the doctor determine which symptoms are relevant. It's important to tell your doctor about your skin condition, headaches, dental problems, fatigue, pain, cough, constipation, problems sleeping, or depression. Many people don't want to "bother" the doctor with what seems to be an irrelevant problem, but since your whole body is experiencing treatment, *everything* is relevant. Some symptoms may be caused by your medications or surgery. Others may indicate an infection that needs to be resolved before treatment can start. Some problems may require a referral to a specialist or to your primary care doctor. Don't try to sort it out yourself; let your oncologist know what's happening.

Bring someone with you to help you remember, ask questions, or take notes. There are many reasons why you could benefit from having someone you trust with you for visits to discuss your treatment plan. You may be anxious, you may not feel well, or you may be fatigued or overwhelmed. Make sure you choose someone who's not so overwhelmed with her own anxiety about your diagnosis or treatment that she would distract you or the doctor from focusing on *your* needs during the visit. That person (spouse, friend, or family member) could act as note taker so that you can concentrate on listening and asking your questions. If you're not effective in explaining the severity or difficulty of a problem, the other person can speak up. After your visit, that person can help you review the visit accurately, since she was there.

Create a system for organizing all the information. People are handing you lots of paper. You should trash some of it, but you'll need to keep some of it. At the end of the day, you'll find that you have lab reports, scan results, phone numbers, lists of questions, insurance forms, drug information, "self-care" handouts, a receipt from the parking garage, and so on. Setting up a filing system for important papers will lower your stress level. Chapter 15 ("Preparing to Start Chemo: A Practical Guide") has many suggestions about how to do that.

A Second Opinion

You may hesitate to seek a second opinion about your treatment plan. You may fear that it would be insulting to your doctor, that your doctor may think that you don't trust him. But seeking a second opinion before starting treatment is very common. Your insurance company may even require it. And remember, your doctor is providing second opinions for other patients all the time.

The benefit of a second opinion may just be to reassure you that the recommended treatment plan is the best for you. If there's a decision to be made about how to proceed, you may benefit from a second opinion, and your doctor may even recommend it. For instance, there may be a choice to make about whether to have radiation or more surgery before or after chemotherapy treatment. You may need to choose from among different combinations of drugs. Or there may be a research study available at another treatment center. Getting a second opinion could help you make these decisions more easily and with more confidence.

First, check with your insurance company to see if seeking a second opinion is a covered benefit, how to have it authorized, and if there are any restrictions about where you can go for this service. Once you know which doctor you'll see for this consultation, check with her office to see what information they need to review before your appointment. Your original oncologist's office may communicate with the consulting doctor's office to help gather the information. When you have your appointment for a second opinion, that doctor may want to examine copies of reports, scans, and slides made from the original tumor. You may have to pick up films or CDs of some tests to bring with you.

Once all the information is gathered, the doctor providing the second opinion can take a fresh look at everything—including you. You'll have another interview and physical examination, and have a chance to ask questions. Your original oncologist will receive a complete report as well.

CLINICAL TRIALS

Researchers are the scientists that develop new and more effective treatments for many diseases. That's how medicine evolves. What we now accept as the standard treatment was once considered experimental. Studies are run by national cancer organizations, government health agencies (like the National Institutes of Health), drug companies, university hospitals, and cancer centers all over the world. They evaluate new drugs, combinations of drugs, and combinations of different kinds of treatments for their effectiveness compared to treatments currently recommended. Results of these studies are then published in medical journals.

Researchers look for something that proves to be *more effective* than standard treatments. They also look for which treatment has the least side effects and is the least disruptive to normal cells. After years of testing and comparing to the standard, a successful treatment then becomes the new standard.

Your doctor may recommend a clinical trial if he thinks that it might benefit you. The new treatment may be more effective in killing cancer cells and preventing their recurrence. It may have fewer side effects or be more convenient (for example, pills rather than IV). The new protocol may mean that you need fewer treatments, or that the treatment may better protect your normal cells or help your body recover faster. Or the trial may show that the standard treatment is as good as or superior to the experimental treatment.

If you're considering being part of a study, you'll be completely informed about the purpose of the study, risks, possible benefits, and possible side effects before you begin. You'll probably have extra blood tests and scans prior to and during your treatment, because the researchers are carefully tracking not only how effective it is at killing cancer cells but also how it's affecting the rest of your body. Often the medication and the research-related testing are provided free of charge.

Phases of Clinical Trials

Each clinical trial goes through a number of phases. When a new drug or treatment is being studied, researchers start by determining its uses, effectiveness, toxicities, and so on. If the drug or treatment shows promise, more studies and trials will be done.

Phase 1: A small number of patients are enrolled initially. This phase evaluates how the drug should be given, how often, and the dose that's effective while causing the fewest side effects.

Phase 2: The drug or treatment continues to be tested for safety and effectiveness for particular cancers.

Phase 3: Larger numbers of people are enrolled for this phase. The new treatment is compared to the standard. A person may be randomly assigned to either the standard treatment or to the new treatment.

Phase 4: This is the surveillance phase, which is done after a new drug or treatment has been approved. It gives more information about its risks, side effects, and who would benefit most from its use.

HOW WILL YOU KNOW IF THE TREATMENT PLAN IS WORKING?

The answer to whether the treatment plan is working depends on a number of factors: the kind of cancer you have, if there's any detectable cancer in your body at the start of your treatment, and if the cancer is causing you to feel ill.

Some people don't have any detectable cancer in their bodies when they start treatment. All the cancer was removed at the time of surgery. They're receiving treatment to eliminate any microscopic spread of cancer cells or growth that doesn't show up in scans or blood tests. So the only indication that the chemotherapy is effective is that the cancer doesn't return. After treatment, they'll continue to have scans and blood tests every few months to assure that they remain cancer free.

For others, the scans or blood tests show the presence of cancer in their bodies even after surgery. The *radiologist*, a physician who specializes in diagnostics, reads these scans and makes precise measurements of the location and size of these areas. When the scans are repeated (usually after several chemotherapy treatments), the doctor looks for the measurement of these areas to be smaller and for these areas to be fewer in number than on the pretreatment scans. Sometimes the areas that previously showed cancer become undetectable after a number of treatments. If the cancer caused an abnormality in your blood tests, your doctor will watch for those tests to return to normal levels as well.

Cancer can make some people feel ill. It can cause pain, pressure, swelling, digestion problems, shortness of breath, and more. Once these people start chemotherapy, they often feel a lot better. So, even without repeat scans, they and their doctors are aware that the treatment plans are working and affecting the source of their symptoms.

TREATMENT PLANS CAN CHANGE

Your doctor will continue to check on your condition throughout the treatment period. She'll monitor your blood counts; digestion; skin; mucous membranes; and how well your lungs, kidneys, liver, and other organs are functioning.

As your doctor continues to monitor your progress, he may determine that a change in your treatment plan is necessary. For instance, it's possible that you'll need a change in the dose or frequency of your treatments. You could need a change in the medications given before or after your treatment to prevent or control nausea, diarrhea, or other side effects. Your doctor may even change to a different chemotherapy medicine if the one you're receiving is ineffective. You may need to change to a new medication because of the side effects you're experiencing or if you develop an allergy to it.

Don't let a change in your treatment plan discourage you; your doctor is fine-tuning the plan so that it's safer and more effective.

IN CONCLUSION

Treatment planning is an ongoing process. It doesn't end when your first chemotherapy begins. Your doctor continues to evaluate the effectiveness of your treatment through physical examination, scans, and blood tests. Your doctor and nurses are constantly evaluating you to be sure that the original plan is working; that you're able to eat, drink, and be active; and that the goals of your treatment are being met.

Chapter 3

Understanding Blood Tests

When you're ill, it seems as if everyone's after your blood. Every time you look up, there's someone in a lab coat, carrying a tourniquet and multicolored test tubes, who needs just a few more ounces. You probably wonder, "Why so many tests? Why so often?" You may even feel that you're giving too much blood and worry about how and when your body will replace it.

You have about four to five quarts of blood in your body, and most blood tests require only about a teaspoon of blood in a test tube. The few teaspoons of blood you lose each time blood is drawn for testing are rapidly replaced. Even someone donating a pint of blood replaces it so quickly that it's possible to donate again in about two weeks.

This chapter covers some of the most frequent blood tests that your doctor may order. Many of them can be done at the same time, with only one needle stick. The nurse or lab technician can simply keep the needle in place and change the collection tubes. Then the samples can be sent to different departments in the lab for analysis. Unfortunately, there are times (especially when you're a patient in the hospital) when, as soon as the lab technician leaves, another comes in for another test and another needle stick. But as a rule, your doctors and nurses try to consolidate the tests to avoid this.

In the hospital, blood for routine blood tests is usually drawn very early in the morning, around five o'clock. This is a source of great annoyance to many people, since they can't imagine why samples must be taken at such an early hour. The reason why blood samples are collected so early is that it takes several hours for the lab to perform all the tests and get the results to the nurses' station and into your chart. When the doctors come each day to review your chart and determine what medications, IVs, treatments, or tests you need, the results of blood tests are an important source of information.

Don't hesitate to ask your nurse or doctor what blood tests are being done and why they're necessary. You also may want to know the results of the tests and what they indicate about your condition. You can also ask for a copy of your blood test results.

WHY TEST YOUR BLOOD?

Blood is the fluid of life. It carries oxygen from your lungs to each and every cell of your body. It supplies the glucose that all your cells need for energy and then carries off the waste products from the cells' activities. Blood contains your body's defense against infection and carries the means of repairing the vessels (arteries and veins) in which it flows. Blood maintains the balance of all the chemicals that are necessary for muscles and nerves to function, and provides the communication and coordination for all your organs to work together. With these diverse functions, you can see why a small sample of your blood provides an amazing window into the health and functioning of every organ. A mere teaspoon or two, when analyzed by the lab, can tell a great deal about you.

Blood is made of cells and plasma. The blood cells are red cells, white cells, and platelets, which are all produced in your bone marrow. The plasma is straw-colored fluid containing blood cells along with glucose, electrolytes, enzymes, minerals, vitamins, hormones, and everything else your body needs to stay alive. A *complete blood count* (*CBC*) identifies the types, quantities, and characteristics of the different cells of your blood. A *blood chemistry* analyzes the plasma.

BONE MARROW: THE BLOOD-CELL FACTORY

Bone marrow is the tissue within your bones where blood cells are made. In infants, all the bone marrow is capable of manufacturing blood cells. But in adults, blood cells are made only in the flat bones, such as the pelvis, sternum (breastbone), vertebrae, and skull.

The bone marrow is like a blood-cell factory. It contains stem cells that have the capacity to evolve into all three types of blood cells. A stem cell can develop into a red blood cell and carry oxygen. Or it can evolve into a white blood cell and fight infection. Or it can evolve into a platelet, which can stop bleeding by forming a clot.

Bone marrow maintains the normal number of the three types of cells by replacing old cells as they naturally die, off and increasing production of any kind of blood cell if there's a special demand for it. For instance, your bone marrow will step up production of white blood cells when you have an infection.

The bone marrow is a place where cells divide very quickly in order to keep up with your body's constant demand for blood cells of all kinds. Since chemotherapy can affect the cells that divide quickly (like cancer cells), it will temporarily affect your bone marrow. Unlike cancer cells, your bone marrow will recover and resume its normal production of blood cells.

Chemotherapy doesn't affect the blood cells that are already circulating in your blood, since they're not dividing. Only the production of new cells in the bone marrow is slowed down. Chemotherapy's effect on your bone marrow usually shows up in your blood-cell count about a week to ten days after your treatment. That's when you can see that the blood cells haven't been replaced at the normal rate. But in another week or so, the number of blood cells in circulation will increase.

Your chemotherapy treatments are timed to allow your bone marrow to recover. Your doctor will always check your blood-cell count before each treatment to be sure that your bone marrow is back on the job of producing blood cells.

RED BLOOD CELLS

Your red blood cells (also called *erythrocytes*) give your blood its color. Ninety percent of each red cell is made up of hemoglobin, a substance rich in iron. The size, shape, and flexibility of red cells enable them to squeeze through the small openings between cells. The red blood cells' purpose is to carry oxygen from your lungs to every corner of your body and carry carbon dioxide from the cells to your lungs to be exhaled. If you have too few red blood cells because of blood loss or because your bone marrow isn't working normally, then your body's ability to carry oxygen and carbon dioxide is jeopardized. This condition is called *anemia*.

When your red-blood-cell count is low, your heart has to work harder to cycle the remaining red cells at a faster rate to provide your body with the oxygen it needs. You may feel tired, since there may not be enough oxygen to keep up with the activity of your muscles. You may feel dizzy when you stand up after you've been sitting or lying down. You may chill more easily or feel more winded after exerting yourself. These are all symptoms indicating that your body needs more oxygen and more red blood cells to carry it.

Red blood cells have a relatively long life span (about three or four months). While the production of new cells may be temporarily slowed down, the fact that they live so long makes the problem much less severe. By the time more cells are needed, your bone marrow has long since recovered and has usually caught up.

A complete blood count (CBC) provides three measurements that reflect the adequacy of your red blood cells. They are the red-blood-cell count (RBC), hemoglobin (Hgb), and hematocrit (Hct).

The *red-blood-cell count* is the number of red blood cells in a cubic millimeter of blood. The normal number of red blood cells is about 4.5 million to 6 million per cubic millimeter for men and 4 million to 5.5 million per cubic millimeter for women.

The *hemoglobin (Hgb) test* measures the amount of this substance in a sample of blood. Hemoglobin is the part of a red blood cell that actually carries the oxygen, so an Hgb test gives a good indication of the cells' ability to carry oxygen from the lungs to all the parts of your body. Normal hemoglobin for men is from 14 to 18 grams per 100 milligrams of blood. For women it's slightly less (12 to 16 grams).

The *hematocrit (Hct) measurement* determines what percent of the sample of whole blood contains red blood cells. Normally, red blood cells comprise 42 to 54 percent for men and 38 to 46 percent for women.

If you've lost a lot of blood or your red-blood-cell production has been slowed down, then all three tests will be lower than normal. As your body increases the production of red blood cells in the bone marrow or you receive a blood transfusion, all three values will rise.

What to Do When Your Red-Blood-Cell Count Is Low

Many people get through chemotherapy without having a significant drop in the production of their red blood cells. Since the cells live for so long and the bone marrow recovers in four to ten days after chemotherapy, they're soon replaced. Depending on your general health, you may be able to cope with a mild drop in red blood cells without noticing anything more than fatigue. The following measures may be helpful:

- Eat a well-balanced diet, especially foods high in iron (like dark-green leafy vegetables and raisins). Drink lots of fluids as well.

- Ask your doctor whether you need an iron supplement.

- Take your time when getting up from a lying or sitting position. If you're dizzy, take some deep breaths until the dizziness subsides.

- Get plenty of rest. During this time, it helps to pace your activities. If you have a lot to do, don't try to get everything done at once. Take breaks to recover your energy before going on.

Stimulating Red-Blood-Cell Production

A special hormone stimulates bone marrow to produce red blood cells. This hormone, *erythropoietin*, is normally produced by the kidneys in response to a drop in the oxygen-carrying capacity of the blood. Erythropoietin works by stimulating the red blood cells to mature faster. A synthetic version of this hormone is available by injection to speed up red-blood-cell production when it has been slowed by the effect of chemotherapy. If you have a severe drop in your red blood cells, you may require a blood transfusion. Your doctor will let you know if either of these treatments could be helpful to you.

WHITE BLOOD CELLS

White blood cells (*leukocytes*) provide your body's defensive response to infection. They're produced and stored in the bone marrow, and released when the body needs them. Once in the bloodstream, they circulate for only about twelve hours. Any inflammation or bacterial invasion will attract these cells, triggering them to leave the bloodstream and gather at the site of infection. There they surround the bacteria or other foreign body, stretching and wrapping themselves around it and then digesting it. White blood cells also help damaged tissue repair itself.

There are five kinds of white blood cells that are produced in the bone marrow. The first three (neutrophils, eosinophils, and basophils) have a granular appearance when seen under a microscope, and thus are called *granulocytes*. The two other types are lymphocytes and monocytes.

Neutrophils. *Neutrophils* are the most numerous white blood cells. They comprise 62 percent of all white blood cells and are the first to gather at an infection. Their job is to localize and neutralize bacteria. Each neutrophil can inactivate from five to twenty bacteria. When neutrophils are used up from fighting bacteria, they rupture, and the contents of the ruptured cell attract even more neutrophils, as well as increase the blood supply to that area. The increased blood circulation can make an infected area appear redder and feel warmer than usual.

Eosinophils. *Eosinophils* are the white blood cells that respond to allergic reactions. Their job is to detoxify foreign proteins before they can harm the body. They also contain toxic granules that can kill invading cells and clean up areas of inflammation.

Basophils. The rarest of the white blood cells, *basophils* release histamine, which increases blood supply and attracts other white blood cells to the infected area. Basophils make it easier for white blood cells to migrate out of the blood into the damaged area. They also release heparin, which dissolves old clots.

Lymphocytes. *Lymphocytes* not only fight infection but also provide you with immunity to certain diseases. For example, the measles virus has an antigen: a substance that your body recognizes as foreign. Lymphocytes react to that foreign substance by forming antibodies. Antibodies are proteins that are designed to kill one specific antigen. There are many kinds of antigens, and your lymphocytes develop many different kinds of antibodies to attack them. These antibodies not only fight the foreign substance but also remember it so that they can kill it whenever you're exposed to it again. Even if it's many years after your first exposure, the antibodies made by your lymphocytes remember the antigen and provide immunity.

Lymphocytes can be produced by the bone marrow or by other organs, such as the lymph glands, spleen, tonsils, and thymus. They move back and forth between your blood and your lymphatic system. While many lymphocytes produce antibodies, others function as regulators for your immune response, either helping it or suppressing it, depending on how well you're fighting an infection.

Monocytes. The last type of white blood cell is the body's second line of defense, because it doesn't respond as quickly as neutrophils. Its job is to move into an infected area to remove damaged or dying cells or cell debris. It contains special enzymes that are very effective at killing bacteria. *Monocytes* are produced in the bone marrow and initially circulate in your blood. Once they leave the blood, they go into the tissue and establish themselves in the lymph nodes, lungs, liver, or spleen.

All five kinds of white blood cells work together to fight infection. The usual signs of infection are swelling, redness, warmth in the affected area, and fever. These symptoms indicate that your immune system is working, fighting bacteria or other foreign organisms. The formation of pus in an infection is really a collection of old, dead bacteria and exhausted white-blood-cell debris.

How Chemotherapy Affects White Blood Cells

Unlike red blood cells, which live for months, white blood cells have a life span of only three or four days, and the bone marrow constantly produces new cells to replace them. It's the bone marrow's production of white blood cells that's most vulnerable to the effects of chemotherapy. The cells that are already in circulation or in your tissues aren't affected because they aren't dividing. But when these cells die off and the reserves have been used up (within a week to ten days after your chemotherapy), your white-blood-cell count reaches its lowest point. This period is called the *nadir*.

The nadir is the time when you're most susceptible to infection. If you're exposed to bacteria during that time, your immune system may not be able to make as strong a response because there are fewer white blood cells to respond. Following the nadir, your bone marrow will begin to catch up with white-blood-cell production and your blood count will recover. Your white-blood-cell count usually recovers by about three weeks after your chemotherapy treatments are over.

Your doctor expects your white blood cell count to drop temporarily, but she'll always check it before you receive your next treatment. If there's a delay in recovery, your doctor may delay your treatment for a few days and then check your blood again. After several chemotherapy treatments, it's not unusual for your white-blood-cell count to be a little slower in recovering.

What to Do When Your White-Blood-Cell Count Is Low

Many people who are getting chemotherapy weather the period when their white-blood-cell counts are low without problem. But you do need to take special precautions to avoid infection during this time. Here's what to do:

- Stay away from anyone who has a cold, the flu, or any infection.

- Stay away from large crowds of people in an enclosed environment to avoid being exposed to coughs and sneezes.

- Keep your skin clean and dry. Moisture provides a breeding place for bacteria.

- Be sure to wash your hands often, especially after using the toilet. Remind others (doctors, nurses, family, and anyone else helping with your care) to wash their hands too.

- Keep your teeth and gums clean, because the food left on your teeth or under your dentures is a place where bacteria could grow.

- Drink plenty of fluids. Urinating frequently will help prevent bladder infections.

- Take special care to wash and disinfect any break in your skin and let your doctor know about any cuts, rashes, or burns. Since it's the action of your white blood cells that causes inflammation, redness, or pus, you may not have these familiar signs of infection while your white-blood-cell count is low.

- Check with your doctor if you have any signs of a cold, cough, flu, or fever during this time as well. He may want you to take an antibiotic to help your body fight infection more effectively.

- Let your doctor know before you go to the dentist, the podiatrist, or any other health care provider. Most invasive procedures should be delayed until your immunity recovers.

When all your chemotherapy treatments are over, your body's defenses will eventually return to normal. But during this time, any possible infection should be treated aggressively.

Stimulating White-Blood-Cell Production

Special proteins in your body called *colony-stimulating factor* (*CSF*) stimulate the production of white blood cells. New techniques in genetic engineering have produced different forms of this protein that can be given by injection to counteract the effects of cancer treatments on the body's immune system. The form of CSF that increases granulocytes is called *G-CSF*. It causes your bone marrow to speed up the maturation and release of those particular white blood cells, shortening the period of time when you're vulnerable to infection.

Not everyone getting chemotherapy will need this medicine to stimulate white-blood-cell production. But if there's a delay in bone-marrow recovery or a high risk of infection, CSF can help your bone marrow recover sooner.

INFECTIONS

You're surrounded by a world you cannot see. All around you are bacteria, molds, yeast, and viruses that can only be observed under a microscope. Everything you touch or eat, and even the lining of your digestive system, is teeming with microorganisms that could cause infection if they were to penetrate into your blood or tissues.

It's your intact skin and mucous membranes that usually keep these microorganisms from invading your blood system. It's only when these natural barriers are compromised that you risk infection. Your immune system then becomes your next line of defense, mobilizing to fight the infection that has penetrated your skin or mucous membranes.

If an infection is severe or your immune system is compromised, you may need some help to fight it. Antibiotics are medicines that help your body fight bacterial infections. There are a number of different antibiotics, and some are more effective in killing certain bacteria than others. Your doctor may want to determine the exact bacteria causing your infection in order to prescribe the best antibiotic. This is done by ordering a culture.

Getting a Culture

You're probably familiar with throat cultures that determine what kind of organism is causing a sore throat. The doctor or nurse takes a sterile swab and wipes the back of your throat with it. Then the swab is smeared across a nutrient-rich gel and placed in a warm environment to encourage the bacteria to grow rapidly. In a day or two, there are enough bacteria growing in the nutrient that they can be examined under a microscope. The microbiologist in the lab can then see the exact bacteria causing the problem and determine which antibiotic will be most effective in killing it. When this test is done, it's called a *culture* (the process of growing the bacteria in a nutrient) and *sensitivity* (the process of determining which antibiotics are most effective in killing those bacteria). Viruses, molds, and yeast can be cultured as well.

Bacteria and other organisms can be cultured from anything your body produces, such as urine, sputum, stool, or drainage from wounds. Blood cultures are quite common. If you have a fever or any other sign of infection, your doctor may want to determine if bacteria (or other organisms) are present in your blood. A sample of your blood is taken and put in an environment that encourages microorganisms to grow. Since your blood supply is so large, it's often difficult to capture a particular organism in a small sample. Accordingly, you may have to have two samples of blood taken a few minutes apart to improve the chances of finding something.

If your infection is severe or your level of infection-fighting white blood cells is low, your doctor may not wait until the exact bacteria have been identified. After a sample of blood has been taken, your doctor may want you to start taking an antibiotic right away. Usually your doctor will choose a *broad-spectrum* antibiotic, named for its capacity to kill many different kinds of bacteria. In a few days, when the lab can identify the exact organism, your antibiotic may be changed to one that's more specific for that organism.

Fine-Tuning the Antibiotic

To fight infections successfully, you need the correct antibiotic at the correct dose for a long enough time to assure that the infection is gone. That's why your doctor and nurse will remind you to take all of the antibiotic prescribed, even if the signs and symptoms of infection seem to disappear after a day or two. Most antibiotic pills are prescribed for a week to ten days. More severe infections may require IV antibiotics for a few days, and then, depending on the organism and your response, you may be switched to pills, tablets, or capsules.

PLATELETS

The cells in your blood that help to form a clot are called *platelets*. Platelets are produced in the bone marrow, from a cell called a *megakaryocyte.*

Platelets help your body stop bleeding from nicks or cuts. They do that by collecting at the site of an injury and making the blood vessel constrict. Platelets then begin a series of chemical reactions that, along with other clotting factors in the liquid part of your blood (plasma), form a clot. After the vessel has healed and the clot has served its purpose, another series of chemical reactions causes the clot to dissolve so that the blood vessel is open again to carry blood.

Platelets are formed in large numbers, with as many as 150,000 to 300,000 in each cubic millimeter of blood. They live for about ten days in circulation. Some chemotherapy slows down platelet production, just as it slows down the production of all the other blood cells that divide frequently. The platelets in circulation are not affected because they aren't dividing, but formation of the megakaryocytes (which will become new platelets) may temporarily fall behind. The period of time when your platelet count is the lowest (the nadir) comes about ten to fourteen days after your chemotherapy.

What to Do When Your Platelet Count Is Low

Many people get through all their chemotherapy treatments without being in danger of serious bleeding because of lack of platelets. Staying safe is mostly a matter of being careful to avoid injury and paying extra attention to any bruise or abrasion.

During the nadir, you may find that you bruise more easily or bleed for slightly longer from a cut or after a blood test. Here are a few recommended precautions:

- Check your skin all over for bruising or broken blood vessels. Check with your doctor if a bruise continues to increase in size.

- Notify your doctor of nosebleeds or headaches.

- Avoid contact sports where you can be injured.

- Wear protective gloves when working in the yard.

- Use an electric razor instead of a blade to avoid cuts or nicks when shaving.

- Notify your doctor if you notice blood in your urine or stool.

- Brush and floss carefully since your mucous membranes are more likely to bleed during this time. Use a soft-bristled brush and a gentle technique.

- Notify your doctor before any dental procedures.

- Notify your doctor before any appointments with other health care providers, including chiropractors, acupuncturists, and podiatrists.

- Avoid any intramuscular (IM) injections. Injections given under the skin (subcutaneous, or SQ) are generally safe, but check with your doctor first.

PLASMA

Plasma is the fluid in which the red cells, white cells, and platelets circulate. It contains many substances that are essential for your body to function. For example, sodium, potassium, chloride, calcium, magnesium, and other elements must be present in your body in specific amounts. That's because salts from these elements, when dissolved, can carry an electric charge that enables your heart, nerves, and muscles to work properly. These elements are called *electrolytes*.

Electrolytes

Your kidneys help to regulate the balance of electrolytes by selectively eliminating or retaining these elements. For example, if you eat food that contains a high level of potassium, sodium, or calcium, your kidneys will keep what's needed and get rid of the excess. Chemotherapy treatments can temporarily affect your body's ability to maintain a normal balance of electrolytes. Your doctor may therefore need to adjust the amount of electrolytes you get in your IV or take by mouth.

Proteins

There are also proteins in plasma. These are large molecules, such as albumin and globulin, whose presence controls the flow of fluid from the blood system to the cells. Low levels of albumin can occur with malnutrition. This may cause water and plasma to leak out of the veins into the surrounding tissue, causing swelling (*edema*).

Enzymes

Your heart and liver contain unique enzymes. If these organs have been damaged (from a heart attack or from liver damage), the enzyme specific to that organ can be detected at higher levels than normal in plasma. When the levels of these enzymes drop back to normal, it indicates that the organ is recovering.

Other Substances in Plasma

The levels of nitrogen, urea, and creatinine found in blood plasma indicate how well your kidneys are working. Since many chemotherapy drugs are excreted through your kidneys, your doctor will check the levels of these substances in your plasma to determine the drugs and the doses that are safe and effective for you.

There are also substances in plasma called *clotting factors*. They work with your platelets to form clots when needed and then work to dissolve the clots when they're no longer needed.

The amounts of glucose, protein, iron, and cholesterol in plasma can reflect your diet or digestion. An analysis of plasma can also provide early warning for diabetes, hormone imbalances, iron and vitamin deficiencies, or the risk of heart disease.

Testing plasma allows your doctor to check on how every organ is functioning. It's important to monitor not only how well the chemotherapy is working to kill cancer cells, but how the chemotherapy is affecting all the normal cells as well.

LOOKING AT YOUR LAB RESULTS

When you look at the printout, you'll see a column or row of abbreviations that indicate the specific blood component tested. Next to that, there's another column or row of numbers that shows each result along with some indication of whether it's higher or lower than the "normal range." (Different labs may have some slight variation in their normal ranges.) As you get used to looking at your lab results, you'll see how these values will change over the weeks of treatment. Your WBC (white blood count) and neutrophils will predictably drop and recover many times over the months of treatment as your body and bone marrow respond to the effects of chemotherapy. You may see some variation in your blood chemistry, such as sodium (Na) or potassium (K), if you have diarrhea or vomiting. You can ask your nurse to help you understand the lab printout and explain the significance of the trends and variations.

TUMOR MARKERS

Research scientists are always looking for a simple blood test that will detect cancer at its earliest stage as well as indicate how well the cancer treatments are working. This kind of test could also warn of recurrence long before there are any symptoms.

Although there's no current blood test that can accurately detect cancer's occurrence or cure, there are a number of substances in your blood whose presence at certain levels is associated with particular kinds of cancers. These substances are called *tumor markers*. Their levels tend to rise if the cancer is growing and drop when the cancer is destroyed.

If you have breast cancer, your doctor may test your blood for the tumor marker CA15-3 or CA27-29. The tumor marker CA-125 may be periodically checked if you have ovarian cancer.

An important drawback of tumor markers is that a rise in the tumor marker is sometimes caused not by cancer but by another disease or condition. A rise in the *prostate-specific antigen (PSA)* can indicate prostate infection as well as prostate cancer. A rise in the blood level of *carcinoembryonic antigen (CEA)* is associated with cancer of the colon, pancreas, breast, or intestines but may also occur with pancreatitis, inflammatory bowel disease, or emphysema.

In other words, tumor markers are not foolproof in their ability to predict the presence or absence of cancer. But they're one of many tools your doctor will use to follow your progress. Comparative X-rays, scans, and physical examinations, along with changes in your tumor markers, are all ways that the doctor can tell how your treatment is progressing.

COMMUNICATING WITH OTHER HEALTH CARE PROFESSIONALS

Let your oncologist know if you're planning any other medical treatments (dentist, podiatrist, or chiropractor) before you go. During the period of time when you have fewer white blood cells or platelets than normal, you're more likely to bruise or bleed easily, and less resistant to infections. Your oncologist will advise you when other treatments are safe and the kind of precautions that other doctors need to take during this time. For the same reason, let other health professionals know that you're receiving chemotherapy so that they'll consider this when planning and scheduling their treatments.

IN CONCLUSION

Blood tests are so common and so useful in the diagnosis and treatment of diseases that medical professionals often forget how stressful they may be for you. Here are some suggestions that may help you get through it:

- It helps if you can relax. If you're not in a panic, your veins are easier to find. Make sure that you're comfortable and that your arm is well supported. When your arm stays still, the needle causes less pain.

- If possible, stay hydrated (continue to drink lots of fluid) before your blood tests so that your veins are full and easier to access.

- If you can anticipate when the test will be done, you may want to ask for a warm blanket to wrap around your arms. The heat will make your veins swell, making it easier for the nurse or technician to take the blood sample.

- When the test is over, apply pressure to the vein for at least five minutes. This is especially important if your platelet count is low and your body takes longer to form a clot. Applying pressure will minimize the amount of bruising and pain you have afterward.

Chapter 4

The IV Experience

Nobody likes needles. No one likes to extend an arm, await the tourniquet, and feel the cold swab of alcohol. You pray that your veins will stand out, and fear that the worried look of the technician indicates that you and your veins might be a problem. People who are receiving chemotherapy have to face that moment of truth many times during their treatments. Frequent blood tests are important to monitor your response to cancer treatments; the recovery of your immune system; how well your kidneys, liver, and other organs are functioning; the presence of infection; and so on. Besides the blood tests, most chemotherapy drugs are given intravenously (in the vein, or "IV" for short). When medicine is sent into your vein, the blood throughout your body quickly distributes it. Many chemotherapy drugs aren't available in a form that you can swallow, because they may damage the lining of your stomach or be rendered less effective by the action of different digestive enzymes and secretions.

THE BASICS ABOUT VEINS

Veins and arteries are muscular tubes that can swell or contract in response to temperature, activity, or emotions. You can notice how prominent your veins get on a hot day or when you're playing baseball or working in the garden. You may have also noticed that your veins seem to disappear when you've been inactive, or when you feel cold or anxious. Unfortunately, many people feel anxious when they're faced with needles while having an IV started or blood drawn. They find that their once-prominent veins are nowhere to be seen. Reducing the circulation to the arms and legs, and instead shunting blood to vital organs is one of the body's involuntary responses to fear.

Fortunately, there are ways of getting veins to dilate and become more accessible. A *tourniquet* (the band that's wrapped tightly around your upper arm) partially constricts the veins and traps some blood in the arm and hand, which makes your veins stand out. Warming your arms and flexing your muscles by clenching and unclenching your fist are other ways you can help your veins fill with blood and stand out.

Good Veins and Bad Veins

The ease or difficulty that a nurse may have in starting your IV depends on a number of factors. The condition of your blood vessels (arteries and veins) reflects your general health and strength. Strong, young, muscular people tend to have strong, muscular blood vessels. Older people, as well as those who are ill or malnourished, have more fragile vessels. Frequent punctures and irritating medications, such as antibiotics and chemotherapy, can make veins temporarily less flexible and more tender and fragile. The skill and experience of the person approaching your veins is, of course, another factor. Starting an IV takes coordination, judgment, and skill. And the more experience that a person has, the fewer problems there will be with the procedure.

Which Vein?

Many different veins can be used to draw blood or start an IV if the veins are sufficiently large and close to the surface, and can be dilated by using a tourniquet. The tourniquet makes the veins easier to feel and see. After the blood sample has been collected or the IV started, the tourniquet is released and normal blood flow returns.

Blood samples are often drawn from a large vein at the inside of your elbow. That vein, however, is rarely used in starting an IV, because it would restrict the movement of your entire arm. In general, the veins in the back of your hand and in the lower arm are best for IVs. They're visible and accessible, and the needle can be anchored (using tape) to prevent accidental removal without restricting your movement.

GETTING YOUR IV STARTED

Your nurse will assess your arm veins carefully by constricting the blood flow with a tourniquet or blood-pressure cuff. Let the nurse know if you have a preference or if there's any restriction about using one of your arms. People who've had lymph nodes removed from under an arm (like many women who've had breast surgery) should avoid using that arm for the IV. That arm may be more vulnerable to infection or the development of swelling (edema). If you're getting a blood test before your chemotherapy treatment, the nurse may first start your IV and then draw blood from the IV line to send to the lab before connecting it to the IV fluid and tubing. That way you avoid having two needle sticks.

The kind of needle used to start an IV depends on whether the IV will be used for a short time (just a few minutes) or over a longer period (several hours or days). Most chemotherapy given in the doctor's office flows into your blood in less than an hour, although you may also get hydrating fluids, other medications (such as nausea-blocking medicines), or both to prevent side effects from the chemo.

Your IV may be started with a *catheter*, a thin, soft tube that lies within your vein, through which fluids and medicines can flow. The catheter is about an inch long and can be attached to a small piece of IV tubing. At first, the catheter covers a thin steel needle. Once the catheter and needle are inserted into the vein, the steel needle is removed, leaving the soft, flexible catheter in place. The catheter is then secured by tape and a small dressing or bandage, which is put over the site where the catheter enters your skin. This catheter may stay in place for up to three days, but it may need to be changed sooner if there's any pain, swelling, redness, or sign of infection.

Right after insertion, you might see a little bit of blood flow back into the tubing attached to the needle. This indicates that the needle is inside the vein. Your nurse also verifies the correct placement of the IV by injecting a small amount of fluid into the needle. The nurse can see that the fluid goes into the vein and not into the surrounding tissue. This shouldn't be painful, and once the needle is inserted and immobilized with tape, there should be no further discomfort. Pain, burning, or swelling is an indication that the needle may not be in the vein or that the vein is leaking. You should tell your nurse immediately if you're having any of these symptoms.

Once the needle is secured and its position is verified, the fluid and medication can be given. It might be given through a syringe directly into the IV tubing. Or it may be diluted with a small amount of fluid from a bottle or plastic bag and dripped through tubing into your vein over a longer period of time. Once again, there should be no pain once the needle is secured.

BAGS, BOTTLES, TUBING, AND PUMPS

IV fluids and medications flow through sterile tubing from a plastic bag or glass bottle. IVs can flow by gravity, with the rate adjusted by a roller clamp on the IV tube. When the fluid or medicine needs to go at a set rate, it can be controlled with a special machine called an *IV pump*. An IV pump can be set at any rate. It also keeps track of how much fluid is left in the bag or bottle and can sense whether there's any resistance to the flow. Resistance may indicate that the catheter is dislodged or the tubing is kinked. The pump also keeps an electronic eye out for any air bubbles in the tubing, and it will make a loud beep to alert you and your nurse if there's a problem. The IV pump is attached to the pole holding the medicines and fluids, and it's plugged into an electrical outlet. It has a built-in battery so that it can be unplugged for short periods of time and still continue to function.

Sometimes two different bags or bottles of fluid will be running simultaneously. For instance, you might have a hydrating solution, which provides water and a small amount of sugar, salts, and minerals. Another bag contains your chemotherapy, which is set to go in at a controlled rate. In addition, other bags might hold one or two IV medications to prevent side effects such as nausea. These may be given both before your chemotherapy and at set intervals during your treatment. There may be times when your IV pole looks like a maze of bottles, tubes, and blinking lights, and you're not sure what's supposed to be dripping! Just ask if you have any questions.

Continuous Infusions

Some chemotherapy medicines are given very slowly over several days. In the past, if you received this type of treatment, it required that you stay in the hospital for the duration of the treatment, although you may not really have needed hospital care. Now there are small, portable IV pumps that are about the size of a transistor radio or a paperback book. These pumps run on batteries and are programmed by your nurse or the pharmacist to deliver the IV medication at the prescribed rate. You can carry the small pump with you in a bag, either over your shoulder or around your waist. That way you can be independent of poles, electrical outlets, and the hospital while getting treatment. The pump is equipped with an alarm to alert you if there's a problem with the machine or the flow of medication. You'll be told how to contact the nurse, clinic, or hospital if problems arise. And they'll tell you when to return to the clinic to have the IV disconnected after the infusion is complete.

STAYING COMFORTABLE DURING CHEMOTHERAPY

Because people receiving chemotherapy often have to sit still for an extended period of time, most clinics have comfortable recliner chairs or beds for them. Bring a sweater or shawl, or ask your nurse for a warm blanket if you get cold. If your waistband, tie, or collar is tight, loosen it. Try to position the arm that has the IV comfortably. Since some chemotherapy medicines leave a metallic taste in your mouth (or your mouth may feel dry from antinausea drugs or anxiety), sucking on hard candy or sipping some water or tea can be helpful. The anti-nausea medications that you may get before your chemotherapy can also make you sleepy. If you feel that way, you may want to doze or listen to music. Some clinics provide CDs or DVDs, or they may have a television you can watch.

Your nurses will let you know what medicines you're getting, what they're for, and how they're likely to make you feel. For instance, some chemotherapy medicines are given with lots of hydrating fluids, and that will cause you to urinate frequently. Some antinausea medicines will make you feel sleepy or forgetful for a few hours. Knowing what to expect will make it all less frightening.

During chemotherapy you should feel no pain or burning. Pain or burning from the IV may indicate that the catheter isn't positioned properly in the vein and that it should be checked or changed. You shouldn't feel nauseated, because you'll probably be given medicines to prevent nausea if the kind of chemotherapy you're getting can cause that problem. Most people get through their chemotherapy treatments without any discomfort, continuing to eat and drink normally. Chapter 5 ("Preventing Nausea") will give you more information about antinausea medicines and provide many self-help tips to avoid this problem.

Staying comfortable, in part, depends on you. Only you can tell how you feel. You're the source of the essential information about what's happening inside your body. If you have nausea, stomach cramps, dizziness, itchiness, or any other unusual symptom, let your nurses know so that they can stop the IV, contact your doctor, and assess the problem. It might take some fine-tuning to get you the medications and doses that will keep you comfortable, but it can and should be done.

HOW DO YOU COPE?

Most nurses who work with chemotherapy have a lot of experience in starting IVs and are very skilled, as well as relaxed and supportive. They know that most of their patients are anxious, especially when first getting chemotherapy. If you're a little stressed out, you aren't the only person receiving treatment who feels this way.

People have different ways of coping with stressful situations. Some people cope by learning everything they can about a new experience. It helps them if they know what will happen, what it will look like, what it will feel like, and what will be expected of them. Others cope by withdrawing into themselves. They don't want a lot of detailed information since it just makes them feel overwhelmed and more anxious. Distraction helps other people. They feel more relaxed if they can focus on something else, like meditation, reading, watching TV, or talking.

Many people say that it helps to have a close friend or relative with them for support. The support can be both physical (holding the person's hand, for instance) and emotional. Having someone to talk to you, distract you, read to you, or just sit quietly with you can make you feel safer and more comfortable in a stressful situation. If you do bring along a support person, be sure that the person knows what you want from her. Talk it over and be specific about what will help you. Do you want a quiet, calm presence, or would you rather have someone distract you with conversation?

What would help you? Take some time to think about how you cope with stress, and then do all the things you can to support your coping style. Would it help you to be familiar with the environment? You can arrange to meet the nurses, see the room where chemotherapy is given, and see other people who are receiving treatment before you start. The nurses can tell you exactly what to expect and how long the process takes, and give you answers to many questions.

While you're getting chemotherapy, your nurses can also be a source of support. Don't forget to communicate to them how they can help. Let them know what your needs are. You might say, "It would help me to know exactly what I can expect. Please explain everything that's happening." Or you might say, "I brought some music with me so I can just space out," or "I'd like my brother to stay with me."

After your first treatment, your anxiety level will probably be much lower. The whole procedure, the environment, and the physical experience will be a little more familiar. You'll also know more about what works and doesn't work to help you relax. Were you able to meditate, or was the room too distracting? Did your sister's chatter help pass the time, or was it annoying? Should you bring that murder mystery to read, or would you prefer leafing through *People* magazine? You'll also know the nurses better and feel more confident about their skills. And they'll know you better and begin to anticipate some of your individual physical and emotional needs.

IV PROBLEMS

It's the moment that everyone fears. Your veins are small, fragile, or invisible. You endure several attempts at starting the IV, and both you and the nurse get more and more tense. What should you do?

Go for the pro. Successfully starting an IV depends a great deal on the skill and experience of the person doing it. And generally, the most skillful people are the ones who do it frequently. In many hospitals, there are special IV teams: nurses who are IV specialists. If you know that you're a "difficult start," you can ask for the IV specialist to see you, or you can ask for the most experienced nurse working that day to start your IV. In time you'll recognize some of the nurses and have more confidence in their ability. Just seeing a familiar face can help you relax, which helps your veins relax as well. Nurses working in outpatient clinics are usually experts in starting IVs. They do it many times a day.

Stay calm. You've probably noticed that when you're anxious, your hands become cold and clammy. That's a normal reaction to fear. Unfortunately, anxiety works against you when you want the veins in your hands and arms to stand out. So anything you can do to lower your anxiety will probably help: deep breathing, having a supportive person with you, meditating, or even just distracting yourself. See Chapter 14 ("Relaxation and Stress Reduction") for more techniques to help you.

Keep warm. Heat causes veins to dilate and fill with blood. That makes starting the IV easier. Your nurse may provide some form of heat for your arms, such as a warm blanket, a heating pad, or a pan of warm water.

Keep drinking. Some people, afraid that they'll feel nauseated from their chemotherapy, don't eat or drink before their treatment. Since antinausea medications are so successful in preventing nausea, this really isn't necessary. In fact, eating and drinking normally will keep your body fluids up and help make your IV easier to start. Your veins will be "fatter" (filled with more blood) if you don't let yourself become dehydrated.

What If Your IV Is Painful?

Sometimes, even if you've been careful not to disturb your IV, the catheter may become dislodged. Then the fluid or medicine, instead of flowing into your bloodstream, begins leaking into the tissue surrounding the vein. The affected area of your arm or hand might start to feel painful, tender, tight, or swollen. You may notice that your ring or watch feels tighter than usual. What should you do?

If you suspect that fluid is leaking out of the vein into the surrounding area, let your nurse know right away. It doesn't matter if it's day or night. The sooner the IV is removed and put into another vein, the better. In the doctor's office, clinic, or hospital, the nurse will watch your vein and the flow of fluid carefully, especially if the chemotherapy medicine is being injected directly into the tubing connected to the needle. Your nurse will frequently check the flow of fluid as well as your arm and vein. He'll ask you if you have pain at the IV needle site. But don't wait to be asked. If you think there's swelling, or if you have any discomfort, let someone know right away.

Even if the catheter or needle is still in place and your vein isn't leaking, your vein may feel irritated. Sometimes diluting the medicine with more fluid or slowing down the rate of the flow helps. Sometimes, however, it's necessary for the nurse to change the IV to another (larger, if possible) vein so that the medicine can be swept along with a faster blood flow.

Monitoring the IV is clearly an important part of your treatment—and your nurse may not always be the first one to notice something. Even though she'll often check your veins and the flow of medicine, it's always helpful for you to stay tuned in at your end.

VENOUS ACCESS DEVICES

Figure 1 shows the veins of the arms and upper chest. The arm veins are called *peripheral veins*, and the blood flow through them is relatively slow compared to the larger veins of the upper chest. All peripheral veins lead to larger and larger veins, which carry a faster blood flow on the way to the heart. Chemotherapy treatments often involve multiple needle sticks for both blood tests and IVs, and can become especially problematic if your arm veins are fragile or small.

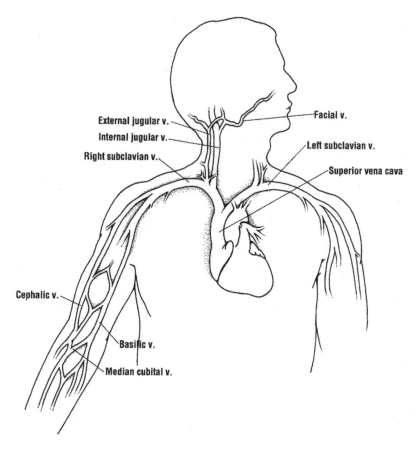

Figure 1

Fortunately, new products have been developed to overcome some of these IV problems. These are called *venous access devices* (*VADs*). They provide a way into the larger veins of your circulation system, where the blood moves more quickly and the effects of medicines and fluid aren't as irritating. VADs eliminate the difficulty of trying to find veins, and they make the process of starting IVs or taking blood tests quick and, in some cases, painless. They can also stay in place indefinitely, without interfering with your normal life at home.

Peripherally Inserted Central Catheters

This device (shown in Figure 2) is called a *peripherally inserted central catheter* (*PICC*), because the catheter is inserted peripherally (into your arm) but travels to a large central vein (in your chest). This kind of IV line is started through a large vein in your arm, either just above or below where your elbow bends. Surgery isn't required. Once your skin is numbed, the flexible IV tube is advanced up your arm vein and through larger and larger veins until the catheter tip is close to your heart, where the blood moves swiftly. An *ultrasound machine* uses sound waves to show your blood vessels and guides the physician or nurse in the proper placement of the PICC. The end of the catheter that emerges from your skin is capped, taped securely, and covered with a sterile dressing. A PICC line can be used for fluids, blood, chemotherapy, and other medications. It can also be used to draw blood for most lab tests. Once in place, there's no need for any needles. The nurse will just remove the cap from the end of the catheter to draw blood, attach it to IV tubing to start your IV infusion, or both. Afterward, the IV line is rinsed and capped again. When you no longer need the PICC (after all your treatments are over), it's easily removed without surgery.

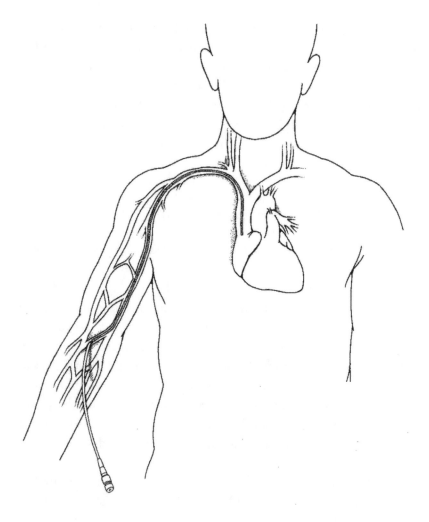

Figure 2

As long as you have this kind of catheter, the place where it emerges from your skin (exit site) will need special care. The dressing must remain clean and dry, and the IV line needs to be rinsed and capped on a regular schedule. If your doctor recommends this kind of IV, your nurse will instruct you on how to care for your PICC at home.

Implanted Vascular Access Devices

An implanted port is another way of accessing the large blood vessels of your body where the blood moves swiftly. One end of the catheter is placed in a large vein near your heart, and the other end of the catheter terminates at the *port*: a small disc, about the size of a quarter, placed under your skin. The center of the port has a raised, rubberlike plug that's self-sealing. A needle can be placed into the port to allow IV fluids (chemotherapy and so on) to infuse or to allow blood to be drawn (for lab tests).

IMPLANTED CHEST PORTS

A physician puts in the port and catheter during a minor surgical procedure. After your skin is numbed, the surgeon makes a small incision below your collarbone and threads the catheter into a large vein. Then he forms a little pocket for the port under the skin of your upper chest (usually near your shoulder). Figure 3 shows an implanted port. The port is about the size of a quarter, and the raised center area is about the size of a nickel. The center area consists of a thick, rubberlike plug that can be punctured with a special needle, which is usually attached to a short piece of IV tubing. Then the IV fluid, blood, or chemotherapy can flow into the port and through the catheter. Once the small incision is healed and the tenderness and minor swelling go away, you should have no pain from the implanted port. Although you'll be able to feel the raised center of the port through your skin, no part of the device is left outside of your skin. You can bathe or swim. No daily care is required, because your own skin protects the catheter from infection.

When you first need to have an IV started or blood drawn, the nurse feels for the location of the raised center of the port, cleans the skin, and punctures through the skin straight into the center plug. Since the center is usually easy to feel, there should be no "fishing around" as there often is with peripheral IVs. Success doesn't depend on your veins. The needle is held securely by the center plug and is much less likely to be dislodged. Once the needle is inserted and secured, the port can be used for all fluids, IV medications, or blood. Most blood tests can be drawn from the same port and needle without any other needle sticks. When your treatment is finished, the catheter is rinsed with a solution that will prevent a clot from forming, and the needle is removed. If you need IV fluid over many days, the needle can stay in place under an occlusive sterile dressing (one that completely covers the entryway) for about a week before it needs changing. Once the needle is removed, the port under your skin automatically seals itself to prevent the bleeding that can sometimes happen when the needle goes directly into a vein.

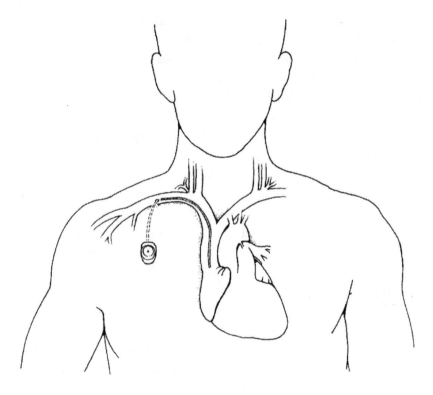

Figure 3

IMPLANTED ARM PORTS

Smaller ports can also be implanted in your arm (shown in Figure 4). As with the PICC, a long catheter travels up a vein in your arm until the catheter tip lies in a large vein of your upper chest near your heart. But instead of having the bottom of the catheter emerge from your arm, it ends in a port, which is implanted under your skin. Once the incision heals, there should be no pain from the port. The entire device is implanted and remains sterile without the need for special cleaning or dressing. And, like the implanted chest port, it will require only a single needle stick to gain access to the blood system.

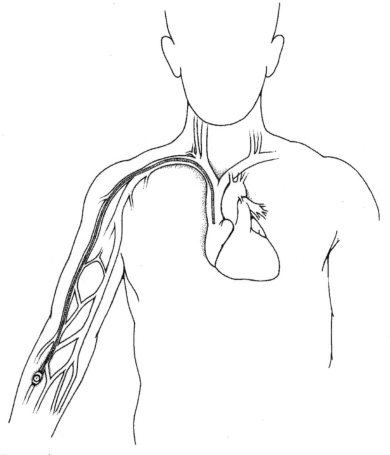

Figure 4

LOCAL ANESTHETICS

If you have an implanted port (whether in your upper chest or in your arm), it means that a needle has to go through your skin. Some people want to have that area numbed to avoid the momentary discomfort of the needle.

In some clinics, the nurse accessing the port may give you a tiny injection of *lidocaine* (a local anesthetic) to numb the skin just before placing the needle. Topical forms of this numbing medication, such as a cream, spray, or patch, are also used to numb the skin over the port so that you don't feel the needle at all. If you're given a prescription for a numbing agent, be sure to read the instructions so that you know when and how to apply it and how long it takes to effectively numb the skin. Your doctor or nurse will give you more information about what options are available at your clinic.

Tunneled Catheters

These catheters are inserted by a surgeon during a minor surgical procedure under local anesthesia. After your skin is numbed, the surgeon makes a small incision near your collarbone and threads the catheter tip into a large vein in your upper chest. A second incision is made several inches away, in the front of your chest. Then the surgeon makes a "tunnel" under your skin between these two incisions. Next, the surgeon will thread the other end of the catheter through the tunnel so that it emerges at about the level of a second or third shirt button.

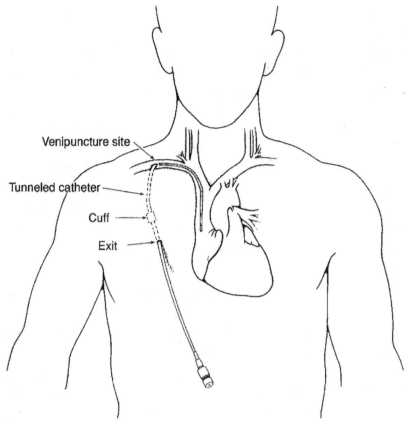

Venipuncture site

Tunneled catheter

Cuff

Exit

Figure 5

Figure 5 shows approximately where the catheter comes out of your body. Because the place where the catheter enters the vein (up by your collarbone) is far away from where it emerges from your skin (midchest), there's less chance of bacteria from your skin causing an infection.

Although there's only one tiny hole in your skin where the catheter emerges, the end of the catheter may split into two or more catheters, or *lumens*, which are capped when not in use. The fluid going into one lumen doesn't mix with the fluid going into the other lumen. This arrangement allows you to get more than one medication at the same time if necessary.

These catheters have a *cuff*, or a wider area along the catheter near the exit site (where the catheter emerges from your chest). You may even feel it under your skin. Your skin will heal around the cuff and hold the catheter in place. This cuff also helps prevent infections from entering the tunnel and traveling up the catheter.

When an IV infusion is started or a blood test is taken, the cap on the line being used can be removed and the catheter attached to an IV line or to a syringe to draw blood.

To prevent an infection, the tunneled catheter will require daily cleaning at the place where the catheter comes out of your skin, and each lumen must be routinely rinsed with special fluid to prevent a blood clot from forming. Your nurse will explain how and when to change the dressing, and how to rinse the lumens and change the caps.

WATCHING OUT FOR PROBLEMS

Most of the time, VADs work well to provide easy access to your blood system so that you can get through your treatment. Your nurses are expert at maintaining the line so that it's free flowing and free from infection. Still, it's always good to know what problems to watch for and how these problems can be resolved.

Possible Infection

The nurses who access your catheter or port will be extremely careful to prevent any contamination that could cause an infection. They do that by using sterile equipment, including gloves and dressings. And they'll constantly assess the skin around the exit site if you have a PICC or tunneled catheter. If you have a port, they'll constantly assess the skin over that area as well. If there's any sign of infection (redness, swelling, pain, drainage, fever, and so on), they'll notify the doctor to evaluate the problem and treat the infection as soon as possible. They may take a sample of any drainage and of the blood within the catheter to send to the lab to identify the kind of bacteria that could be causing the problem. You may be given antibiotics to fight the infection. In some cases, the catheter may need to be replaced.

Even though your nurse and doctor will be watching carefully, you may be the first one who notices a change that may indicate the start of an infection. If this happens, call the clinic and let them know your concern. The earlier an infection is treated, the better.

Keeping the Catheter Free Flowing

Anything that blocks the catheter will mean that fluid can't freely flow through the catheter and blood can't be drawn out of it.

After each use, your VAD will always be completely rinsed to clear the catheter of all blood or medications. Finally, it's rinsed again with a special solution that prevents a clot from forming within it. Sometimes, if the catheter doesn't allow blood to flow out (for blood tests), it may just be a "positioning" problem. The catheter tip may be right up against the wall of the blood vessel and may not allow blood to flow freely. Your nurse may have you change positions, cough, or raise your arms so that the tip of the catheter moves slightly within the blood vessel and the problem is solved.

If the catheter still doesn't flow freely, it may be because a clot has formed within or around the catheter. If that happens, your nurse may instill a clot-dissolving medicine into the catheter, which is usually successful in melting the clot. In a few minutes the catheter is free flowing again. If the problem persists, your doctor may send you for a "dye" study in the X-ray department. There they inject the catheter with a radio-opaque dye that shows up on an X-ray. That way they can check whether the catheter is intact and in the right place within your blood vessel, or whether a clot has formed.

Circulation Problems

If a clot does form around the catheter where it lies within the vein, it may impede the flow of blood through that vein. This can cause swelling in your arm, shoulder, chest, or neck on the side where you have the VAD. At first you may find that your ring or watch is tight, or you may see or feel tightness in your skin. You may be the first to notice the changes, and it's important to call the clinic to let your doctor know about your concern so that it can be treated right away. You may be sent for an ultrasound test that uses sound waves to assess the circulation in the blood vessels of your arm and upper chest. If a clot is causing the problem, you'll be given medicine that will melt the clot and restore normal circulation.

WHICH ONE IS RIGHT FOR YOU?

Not everyone will need a central line, a tunneled catheter, or an implanted port. There are many, many people who complete chemotherapy treatment and blood tests without needing any such device. Their veins can tolerate the kind of medications and fluid they need. Although it's never pleasant to have IVs started or blood drawn, they get through it without major problems. If you need a VAD, you and your doctor and nurse will discuss the risks and benefits of each one. Your doctor will consider the kind of chemotherapy you need, your veins, and your preference. You'll be able to see what each device looks like and perhaps talk to someone who has one.

Although it's not easy to face the minor surgery that's needed to have a VAD put in your body, once it's in place, many people experience it as a great relief. Their IVs are easily started, blood tests are easily obtained, and their arms and hands are freer while they get treatment.

IN CONCLUSION

For many people, a good deal of dread and fear about getting chemotherapy is associated with the frequent blood tests and IVs. They may feel out of control when their veins won't cooperate and getting an IV started becomes difficult. In time you'll find your own unique ways of relaxing and coping during this stressful period. Hopefully, you'll come to trust the skill and support of the people who are caring for you. Just knowing what to expect, what's happening, and what it will feel like can make it all less overwhelming.

Chapter 5

Preventing Nausea

Of the possible side effects of cancer treatments, people often say they dread nausea and vomiting the most. They may have known someone who received chemotherapy or radiation therapy and suffered severe nausea without effective antinausea medication. Or they may recall times during their own lives when they were nauseated, and remember how debilitating it was.

It's a misconception that people who receive cancer-fighting treatments such as chemotherapy suffer continuous, unrelieved nausea and vomiting. First, it's important to remember that not all cancer-fighting treatments cause severe nausea. Some may cause mild nausea or no nausea at all. Second, nausea caused by chemotherapy usually lasts for a limited amount of time (from two to forty-eight hours for most chemotherapy drugs). Third, extensive research has led to the development of new medications that can prevent or relieve the nausea associated with cancer treatments.

WHAT CAUSES NAUSEA?

There's actually an area in your brain that, when stimulated, causes the feeling of nausea. It's called the *chemoreceptor trigger zone* (*CTZ*), and it lies in the center of your brain. This area may be stimulated by a number of different events. The CTZ may be stimulated by a feeling of fullness in your stomach (from too much pizza and beer, for example), or it may be stimulated by dizziness (seasickness or motion sickness). Certain sights, odors, or thoughts may cause nausea as well. Some people may feel nauseated and even vomit from anxiety, fear, stage fright, unpleasant odors, the sight of blood, or the thought of getting an injection.

NAUSEA AND CHEMOTHERAPY

The CTZ is sensitive to the chemicals in your body. Some chemotherapy drugs make your body release other chemicals, such as dopamine and serotonin, which can stimulate the CTZ. Every chemotherapy drug has been rated as to its *emetic potential*: the chances that it will cause you to feel nauseated or to vomit. Some drugs rarely cause nausea (meaning that without antinausea medication, fewer than 30 percent of people will feel nauseated from that drug). Some chemotherapy medicines are considered only moderately nauseating. And then there are some that will very likely make you feel nauseated unless you're given medication to prevent it. So, right from the beginning, your doctor can tell you if nausea will likely be a problem.

Another factor that may determine how nauseated you feel is the dose. A chemotherapy drug may not cause nausea at a low dose, but it may cause the problem at higher doses or when given in combination with other, more nauseating drugs.

There are always individual differences in how people react to any treatment. Some people are just more likely to feel nauseated, just as there are some people who are more likely to suffer morning sickness or motion sickness. Your doctor may try to predict how much of a problem nausea will be, but you may be less or more nauseated than expected. The key is to work with your doctor and nurse to determine the type and the amount of antinausea medication you need to prevent or minimize the problem.

TYPES OF ANTINAUSEA MEDICINES AND HOW THEY WORK

The stimulus that triggers nausea can come from different places in your body: the stomach, the inner ear, even sensations and thoughts, as well as chemicals or radiation. To prevent or relieve nausea, different drugs work in different ways. Some drugs prevent nausea by blocking the body's release of histamine, dopamine, or serotonin so that the CTZ won't be stimulated. Some drugs speed up the passage of food through the digestive system so that your stomach empties quickly and there's less fullness to stimulate the CTZ. Some drugs prevent or relieve the feeling of "acid stomach." Other medications help you relax and even sleep through the period of time when you're most likely to feel nauseated.

Keep in mind that whether or not you become nauseated from chemotherapy doesn't indicate whether the treatments are working. And getting medications to prevent or relieve the nausea doesn't make the treatments less effective.

The following drugs are commonly used to prevent nausea during chemotherapy. The generic name is given first, followed by the brand name(s) that may be more familiar to you. Next comes a general discussion of how each drug works and some side effects to watch out for.

Medications to Prevent Nausea

There's a group of medicines that can block the receptors in the CTZ and the stomach so that they won't be affected by chemicals that your body produces in response to chemo. These medicines have made it possible to effectively prevent or control nausea associated with even the most nauseating cancer-fighting treatments.

Some receptor-blocking medicines work by preventing *serotonin* (a chemical released by your body in response to chemotherapy) from getting through to the 5HT3 receptors and causing nausea. They're known as *5HT3 antagonists* or *serotonin blockers.*

Ondansetron (Zofran), granisetron (Kytril), and dolasetron (Anzemet) are examples of serotonin-blocking medicines. They all work in a similar way. These medicines are given by IV or in a pill form before chemotherapy, and the effect will last for about twelve to twenty-four hours. If nausea is likely to last longer than twenty-four hours, you'll be given a prescription for this kind of medication, which you can take at home for the next one to two days. Your doctor or nurse will let you know how many days and how often to take these nausea-blocking pills.

Palonosetron (Aloxi) is another medication that works the same way, but the nausea-blocking effects can last up to five days. Given by IV, it's most effective if provided during the first two days after chemo.

One downside of these medicines is that they can cause constipation. To prevent this problem, you should increase your fluids. Some people take a stool softener on the days they take this drug. You may also need to take a laxative if you don't have a bowel movement after a day or so. These drugs can also cause you to have a headache. Ask your doctor or nurse for a pain reliever or a different nausea-blocking medicine if you have this symptom.

Another kind of nausea-blocking medicine works by blocking *substance P* (a chemical released by your body in response to chemotherapy). Known as an *NK1 antagonist*, it blocks substance P from getting through to the NK1 receptor in the CTZ and causing nausea.

Aprepitant (Emend) is an example of this kind of nausea blocker. It's given before your treatment by IV or by pill. The pills come in two different strengths. You take the larger dose just before your chemotherapy. The nausea-blocking effect lasts for about twenty-four hours. For the next two days (after your treatment), you take a smaller dose of Emend to continue blocking nausea. The nausea-blocking effect can last up to five days.

If you have a prescription for Emend, have it filled at the pharmacy and bring it with you to the clinic. After your labs are checked and you know for sure that you're getting treatment, then you can take the first Emend pill. That way, if your treatment is delayed for any reason, you don't waste it or take it unnecessarily.

Medications to Relieve Nausea

The drugs described in the previous section are used to prevent nausea. If they're not completely effective, the following drugs can be used to relieve nausea when it occurs.

Steroids like dexamethasone (Decadron and Hexadrol). It's not known exactly how steroids work to prevent nausea. It's possible that they prevent the chemicals that are released by the body in response to chemotherapy from getting through to the CTZ and therefore make it less likely that you'll feel nauseated. This kind of drug is usually given by IV or orally *before* treatment in combination with other antinausea medicines.

Your doctor may also want you to take a small dose of Decadron by pill for a few days *after* chemo. Decadron seems to help the nausea-blocking medicines work better. It's very effective in relieving delayed nausea or queasiness that can persist for up to a week.

Side effects to watch for are water retention, restlessness, confusion, insomnia, and euphoria (feeling "high"). Steroids can also increase your appetite or cause your skin to flush. People who have diabetes need to be aware that steroids can cause a temporary elevation in blood sugar. Steroids taken orally can be irritating to the lining of the stomach, and that in itself can cause nausea. Always take steroid pills with food to prevent stomach irritation.

Prochlorperazine (Compazine). This drug was the mainstay of antinausea treatment for many years before the nausea-blocking medicines were developed. It acts in the CTZ by blocking dopamine receptors. Dopamine is released by the body in response to some chemotherapy drugs and can cause nausea. Compazine can be used alone for preventing nausea when you're getting mildly nauseating chemotherapy. It's available in many forms, including a pill, a long-acting capsule, a rectal suppository, an injection in the muscle, or by IV.

Side effects to watch for are drowsiness (don't drive) and low blood pressure (usually only a problem if given by IV). In some people, Compazine may also cause an uncomfortable jittery feeling or restlessness. This reaction is called *akathesia*, and it goes away if you take a mild tranquilizer such as diazepam (Valium) or lorazepam (Ativan). If you're having any side effects, be sure to call your doctor to see if she wants you to change to a different medication or to take something to counteract these symptoms.

Lorazepam (Ativan). This drug is a tranquilizer in the same family as Valium. It doesn't block dopamine at the CTZ or speed up the digestive tract but works by making you relaxed, forgetful, and sleepy. It's sometimes used alone, but often it's used in combination with other antinausea drugs if you're getting moderately to highly nauseating chemotherapy, or if you're feeling nauseated from anxiety associated with chemotherapy. You can take this drug by mouth, by injection in the muscle, or by IV. The nongeneric (brand name) form of this drug (Ativan) is easily absorbed under the tongue through the mucous membranes. This is particularly helpful if you're vomiting or having difficulty swallowing pills because of nausea.

The side effects to watch for are sedation and forgetfulness. Do not drive when taking this drug. It may also cause unsteadiness, weakness, or a mild lowering of blood pressure. Call your doctor if these side effects are a problem. You may need to use a smaller dose, take it less often, or change to a different medication. Taken at night, lorazepam can help you fall asleep as well as relieve nausea.

Other Medications That Can Help

There are other drugs your doctor may recommend in combination with those listed above. For instance, metoclopramide (Reglan) helps the stomach empty quickly by speeding up the digestive tract. It's effective in relieving nausea as well as the feeling of being overfull after eating a small amount. You wouldn't use it if you also have diarrhea, because in that case the digestive system may already be moving things out too quickly.

Antihistamines such as diphenhydramine (Benadryl) are useful in preventing nausea associated with motion sickness. When used with other antinausea medications, Benadryl can make them even more effective.

Some people may get some benefit from smoking marijuana or taking the drug dronabinol (Marinol), which contains the active ingredient in marijuana. In combination with other antinausea medications, it can help prevent nausea as well as stimulate your appetite.

Drugs that neutralize or decrease stomach acid (Pepcid, Prilosec, Tagamet, Zantac, Aciphex, Protonix, and so on) can also help to prevent or relieve nausea when used with other antinausea drugs.

Every medicine has potential side effects. To be safe, always consult with your doctor or nurse before taking any new medicines—even ones you can buy over the counter (without a prescription). They can give you guidance about which medications would be most effective, how and when to use them, and any reason *not* to take them. Don't try to do it on your own.

PATTERNS OF NAUSEA

These days it's unusual for anyone to experience nausea during treatment. That's because if you're getting chemo that's likely to cause nausea, you'll be given medication that will prevent nausea even before the chemo is started. Most people are comfortable during treatment: able to eat, drink, talk, and read. If the chemotherapy is likely to cause nausea for longer than twenty-four hours, you'll be given a prescription for medications to take at home to continue to prevent it. Your doctor or nurse will give you a schedule instructing you how and when to take these medications. The specific medicines will vary depending on what chemo drug you're getting and the dose and frequency, as well as your own sensitivity.

Breakthrough Nausea

Even when given the nausea-blocking medicines before and after chemotherapy, some people have periods when they still feel slightly nauseated or queasy, or even vomit. That's why your doctor will give you a prescription for something you can take to turn off that problem. That's sometimes referred to as "rescue" antinausea medicine. Prochlorperazine (Compazine), lorazepam (Ativan), or metoclopramide (Reglan) can possibly give you immediate relief.

It's important to take something at the first sign of breakthrough nausea. You want to keep the problem from getting worse. Don't wait for it to pass. Take one of the rescue medications at the first sign of any nausea. It's easier to control and relieve nausea when it's still mild than when it might become more severe and possibly cause you to vomit. Short-acting rescue medicine is meant to be taken as often as necessary (following the directions on the label). Your doctor will give you specific guidelines about when and how often to use these medications. The rescue meds are not intended to replace the nausea-blocking medicine, which is usually taken on a set schedule.

If you need to take the rescue medicine several times during the day because of breakthrough nausea, let your doctor or nurse know. They may want to change to another nausea-blocking medicine that will be more effective and give you greater relief.

Delayed Nausea

If your nausea persists beyond the three to four days after treatment, this is called *delayed nausea*. It's important to get relief from this so that you can continue to eat and drink, and be active and comfortable. At this point the CTZ is probably not being stimulated by serotonin or other nausea-inducing chemicals your body produces in response to the chemo, so the nausea-blocking medicines (5HT3 antagonists) probably won't be as effective as they were the first few days after your treatment. You can get better nausea relief by using other drugs, such as dexamethasone (Decadron), metoclopramide (Reglan), and prochlorperazine (Compazine).

Nausea from Anticipation

You may develop nausea that's not directly caused by the chemotherapy. Some people who suffer unrelieved nausea from cancer treatments begin to automatically associate the treatments with feeling nauseated. This is a conditioned response to a strongly unpleasant experience. As a result, anything associated with the treatment may trigger this reaction: the ride to the office or hospital, the sight of the nurse, the IV tubing, the smell of alcohol. This phenomenon of feeling nauseated without a physical reason is called *anticipatory nausea and vomiting (ANV)*. The best treatment for ANV is prevention. If you didn't suffer significant nausea with one treatment, then you won't likely anticipate feeling nauseated with the next one.

Anxiety also contributes to nausea, especially nausea from anticipation. Some people avoid pretreatment jitters and nausea by taking antinausea medication even before they leave the house. Or, if they have to drive, they may take the pill immediately after arriving for their appointments. The medication that seems to work best for ANV is lorazepam (Ativan), but anything that allows you to relax can help prevent nausea. Acupuncture or acupressure treatments by skilled and experienced practitioners have been shown to be very effective in controlling and relieving nausea, especially nausea triggered by anxiety.

The following are a few more suggestions to lower the anxiety that may contribute to nausea. They're covered in more detail in chapter 14, "Relaxation and Stress Reduction."

Progressive muscle relaxation (PMR) is a way of counteracting anxiety by learning to relax all the muscles of your body. Then you can use visualization to psychologically remove yourself from a stressful environment.

In addition to PMR, other relaxation techniques that may prove useful in relieving anticipatory nausea are explained in chapter 14. Deep breathing, healing imagery, mindfulness, imagery, and self-hypnosis are also excellent ways to lower your anxiety. Sometimes just bringing a book or magazine to glance through may distract you. Some people find that bringing a friend to sit and chat, or listening to some music with headphones is helpful to feel less anxious and lessen the chance of developing anticipatory nausea.

THE IMPORTANCE OF FLUIDS

Everything that you take by mouth (food, fluid, medication, and so on) eventually enters your bloodstream, where it circulates through your entire body. Waste products are filtered from the blood by the liver or kidneys and are eliminated in the urine and stool. The more fluids you take in, the easier it is for your body to break down the chemical by-products and eliminate them.

Staying well hydrated after chemo has many benefits. Dying tumor cells release chemical waste products after chemotherapy that can cause nausea, and drinking fluids helps wash them away. Some chemotherapy drugs can damage the bladder or kidneys if you're not able to drink lots of fluids and urinate frequently. Some of the nausea-blocking medications can cause constipation, and drinking plenty of fluids can help prevent that problem.

One of the dangers of continuous nausea and vomiting is that it makes it difficult to take fluids by mouth. When you're in the hospital or clinic, you'll probably receive fluids directly into your bloodstream by IV. But when you're at home, after your treatment or after a stay in the hospital, it's especially important to control nausea so that you can drink. If you're too nauseated to drink, you may become dry or dehydrated. When you're dry, the nausea may get worse. The result is a vicious cycle. Unrelieved nausea causes dehydration, which intensifies the nausea. Preventing that cycle is essential.

What Is Dehydration?

If you haven't been able to drink because of nausea, or if you've been vomiting a great deal, you'll feel dry. Your mouth and lips will be dry and may be flaky or cracked. Your blood pressure may be lower than usual, and you may feel dizzy when first standing up. (Note that since some antinausea medicines can cause dry mouth and slight dizziness, those symptoms may not necessarily mean that you're dehydrated.) When you're dehydrated, your body will try to hold onto all the fluid it can, so you'll notice that you're urinating less frequently and that the volume of urine is less than usual. Your urine may appear darker because it's more concentrated. You may notice that your weight is down several pounds from before you had your treatment. These are all signs of dehydration.

What to Do If You Are Becoming Dehydrated

Be sure that you take the antinausea medication prescribed. If you're vomiting and can't keep pills down, call your doctor for advice. After taking the medication, wait about half an hour and then try sips of fluid. Any kind of fluid is fine: water, tea, Popsicles, or broth. Drink a small amount frequently (try half a cup every half hour). At first you may be able to tolerate only water, but once you feel a little better, try taking in fluids that have calories, such as soda, diluted fruit juice, Popsicles, and tea with honey. You need some calories or you'll feel very weak. Add easily digested solid food cautiously. You may be able to tolerate a little sherbet, applesauce, or toast. See chapter 7 ("Maintaining Good Nutrition") for more suggestions on how and what to eat when coping with nausea.

Keep track of how much fluid you're drinking and how often you vomit, as well as how often you urinate. If you're still nauseated and think you may be getting dehydrated, call your doctor. Don't wait until you're severely dehydrated to call. Be sure to supply the kind of information that will enable your doctor to accurately evaluate your condition. Tell the doctor:

- How much fluid you drank in the last twenty-four hours

- How often and approximately how much you've vomited in the last twenty-four hours

- What antinausea medicines have been prescribed, whether or not you've taken them, how well they worked, and what problems, if any, they've caused

- How often and approximately how much you have urinated and if your urine appears dark (some chemotherapy medicines will discolor your urine for a few hours, so it may be difficult to tell if your urine appears darker than normal due to dehydration)

- If you've lost weight since getting your treatment (weigh yourself before you call)

- If your mouth, lips, and skin feel dry

- If and when you feel dizzy (does it happen all the time or just when first rising from a sitting or lying position?)

Also let your doctor know if you have other symptoms that are affecting your condition, such as:

- If you have a fever (take your temperature before calling)

- If you have pain: where, how long it lasts, what makes it better or worse

- If you are diabetic (check your blood sugar before calling)

- If you have missed taking other medications because of the nausea or vomiting (heart or blood-pressure medication, anticonvulsants, pain medication, hormones, steroids, and so on)

- If you have other digestion problems, such as diarrhea, heartburn, or bloating

Your doctor may want you to come into the office or clinic to check your blood pressure and test your blood to see how dehydrated you may have become. It may be necessary to give you extra fluids and antinausea medications by IV as well as to make changes in the medications you take at home. Dehydration is a temporary condition that's usually corrected quickly with replaced fluids and medicines.

STEP-BY-STEP HINTS

Here are some suggestions to help you get through your chemotherapy treatment. By preventing nausea you can be comfortable, stay well nourished, and feel better sooner.

Before Treatment

It's not necessary to have an empty stomach before getting chemotherapy. Staying well nourished and well hydrated (drinking lots of fluids) will help you feel stronger and help your body eliminate waste products more quickly. Eat and drink regularly until about two hours before your treatment. Eat foods that are easily digested (high carbohydrate, low fat). Stay away from spicy food or food that will give you a lingering aftertaste that may make you feel nauseated later (onions, garlic, and so on). Your doctor may want you to take antinausea medicine before coming to the clinic or hospital.

During Treatment

Do whatever you can to lower your anxiety. Bring a book, music, a CD, or a friend to occupy you while you're waiting for treatment. Some antinausea medicine might make you feel sleepy, so sleeping through longer chemotherapy treatments might be possible. Wear comfortable clothes, loosen your belt or tie, and bring a sweater or ask for a blanket if you feel cold. Some chemotherapy drugs leave a metallic or unpleasant taste in your mouth, so sucking on hard candy or chewing gum might help.

After Treatment

There are a number of things you can do to prevent nausea during the first few days after treatment. It's important to let your doctor or nurses know if you're experiencing unrelieved nausea or any troublesome side effects from the chemo or antinausea medicines, or having difficulty eating, drinking, sleeping, and so on. Chapter 7 ("Maintaining Good Nutrition") has additional important information about how to manage your food and fluid intake during this time.

MEDICATIONS

Start by taking the medication in the dose and frequency recommended. For instance, if you're getting a kind of chemotherapy that has very little chance of causing nausea, your doctor might recommend taking nausea-relieving medicine only if you experience that problem. Be sure to let your doctor know how often you needed it and whether it was effective.

If you're getting chemotherapy that's more likely to cause nausea, you may be given both nausea-blocking and nausea-rescue medications to take at specific times for the first few days after treatment. Then there may be a different combination of medicines that will relieve delayed nausea if the problem continues.

Be alert to any side effects that may occur, and notify your doctor or nurse as soon as possible if you have any problems. Remember, everyone has his own unique responses to treatment and to the antinausea medicines. Your doctor needs your feedback to make adjustments in the plan so that it works for you. You may need to change to a different medication. You may need to change the schedule, the dose, or the frequency of the medication, or you may need to add another medication to counteract a bothersome side effect.

FOOD AND FLUIDS

Eat small amounts, more frequently. Avoid feeling overfull. Eat bland foods (mashed potatoes, cottage cheese, toast, sherbet, crackers).

You may be very sensitive to the way foods smell. Foods that are served cold or at room temperature have fewer aromas. Stay out of the kitchen as much as possible. Prepare dishes for yourself or the family that are quick and easy with minimal sights or odors that may upset you.

If you're diabetic, you have to be careful that the medication you take to control your blood sugar is appropriate for how much you eat. You might need to check your blood sugar several times on the day of your treatment to make sure it doesn't get too low or too high. Your doctor may want to adjust your insulin dose or other blood-sugar medication until you can eat normally.

Sometimes sweet juices are hard to tolerate after treatment. If that's true for you, try lemonade, broth, club soda, or ice water. Try mixing a little juice with mineral water. You might need to try several different kinds of tastes before you discover what works best.

It's most important to drink fluids. Don't worry if, at first, you don't feel like eating solid foods. Try Popsicles, tea, juices, soup, soda, watermelon, or ice. Drinking with your meal may make you feel over-full and bloated, so drink fluids before or after eating solid food. Drink small amounts of fluids frequently to avoid feeling too full.

Rinse your mouth or brush your teeth before and after eating to avoid lingering tastes that may be nauseating.

ACTIVITIES

Fresh air and mild physical activity help prevent nausea. Take a walk or sit on the porch or by an open window. Distractions may help. Go to the movies, read a book, talk to a friend, listen to music, or play cards.

SLEEP

Some antinausea medications may make you sleepy. If you're supposed to take a medication on a set schedule during the day, you may want to set the alarm clock so that you can wake up, take the medication, and then go back to sleep. If you aren't scheduled to take antinausea medication in the middle of the night, then take it when you first wake up—before you get out of bed and start moving around.

RELAXATION

If you feel anxious, relaxing may be easier said than done. There are a number of CDs and DVDs that you may find useful to help you clear your mind and relax every muscle in your body. You may find that the tension you hold in your face and jaw or in your shoulders or abdominal muscles is adding to your anxiety or feelings of queasiness. Some CDs or DVDs provide peaceful and relaxing images and music. After you practice with these aids for a period of time, you may be able to relax yourself very quickly with or without them anytime you feel tense or anxious.

SELF-TALK

The things you say and think to yourself can either help you cope or cause you more stress. Many of these thoughts are unconscious and so automatic that you may not even be aware of them. Pay attention and try to tune in to what you may be saying to yourself that increases your stress and worries about nausea (or any other scary symptom). It may help to write these thoughts down. This makes them more conscious and more manageable. It also allows you to argue against them and replace these anxiety-provoking thoughts with thoughts that are supportive, accurate, and focused on coping.

Your anxiety-producing thoughts may sound like this:

- I can't stand it; this is too much.

- I feel so helpless; there's nothing I can do.

- The antinausea medicine isn't working; nothing will help.

- I'll never feel any better.

You can replace these anxious thoughts with supportive thoughts that help you cope:

- I can get through this. The discomfort will only last a few hours.

- If this medicine isn't working to relieve my nausea, there are other medicines that I can try.

- The chemotherapy is effective, no matter how nauseated I feel.

- I'm learning how my body reacts to chemotherapy and to the antinausea medicines.

- I am in charge; I can take the medicine that I need in order to feel better.

- It's okay to sleep and let the hours pass.

- The kids (or spouse or job) are taken care of for now. Right now I can pay attention to me and take care of myself.

- I know how to relax, distract myself, and feel better.

- I know that _____ is here for me if I need him or her.

Write down your own coping thoughts. When you find your anxiety rising, tune in to what you're silently saying to yourself and talk back, using the coping statements that help you feel better.

IN CONCLUSION

Nausea and vomiting can be very debilitating, both physically and emotionally. Fortunately, there are strong and effective medications and relaxation techniques that really work. Lots of people get through chemotherapy treatment with minimal nausea or no nausea at all. That's the goal: to get through this time and remain comfortable, well nourished, well hydrated, and able to perform the normal activities of your life as soon as possible. This is possible only if side effects like nausea and vomiting are controlled.

Chapter 6

Coping with Other Digestion Changes

When people think about the side effects of chemotherapy, nausea and vomiting are the symptoms that most frequently come to mind. But other parts of the digestive system can be affected as well. Unlike nausea, which is usually associated with the period of time immediately following treatment, other digestive-system side effects may not happen until a week or two later.

Chemotherapy often affects cells that frequently divide; these include the cells lining your entire digestive system. Normally, those surface cells that are old or dying are continually replaced by new cells. But if there's a delay in the replacement of old cells because of the effects of chemotherapy, you can develop problems such as a sore mouth and throat, taste changes, and diarrhea or constipation. This chapter discusses these and other side effects that can temporarily affect your digestive system, why these side effects occur, and what you can do to feel better.

As with any side effect caused by cancer treatments, the chance of developing the problem and the severity of the problem are related not only to the type of medication or treatment, but also to the dose and your general health and age. Some chemotherapy medicines affect your digestive system more than others. If you're getting radiation therapy at the same time as chemotherapy, you're more likely to have digestive problems if the radiation field includes your digestive system.

Your oncologist and nurse will let you know how your treatment may affect your digestive system and what you can do to prevent or manage any problems.

YOUR DIGESTIVE SYSTEM

To visualize the way food travels through your body, you might think of a large tube. This tube starts at your mouth and ends at your rectum. The mouth is the place where the digestion of food and fluids starts. When you chew, the food is mixed with saliva, which begins to break down the food into substances the body can use.

When you swallow, the food and fluids travel down a long, straight section of the tube called the *esophagus*, which connects to your stomach. Once in the stomach, food is further broken down by the mechanical action of muscles churning and by the chemical action of digestive enzymes found in stomach acid.

The partially digested food moves from your stomach into your small intestine, which is approximately twenty-one feet long. Because it's so long and the space in your abdomen is fairly compact, the intestine winds back and forth in your abdominal cavity like a ribbon. It is in your small intestine that most of the nutrients are absorbed into your bloodstream.

What remains of food after digestion are waste products. These move into the large intestine (also known as the *colon*). Your colon is about five feet in length and ends with your rectum. As the waste products move through the large intestine, fluid is absorbed into your blood system. By the time the waste products have traveled through the entire colon and are ready to be eliminated from your body, the stool is no longer liquid, but a formed solid.

Chemotherapy can cause problems at various points in the digestive system. Let's take a look at each of them.

MOUTH AND THROAT PROBLEMS

Since chemotherapy can temporarily affect the cells of your mouth and throat, it's possible to have a dry or sore mouth or throat, taste changes, or infection.

Dry Mouth

There may be times during chemo when your mouth feels dry, you have less saliva, or your saliva is thick. Some of the medicines you take may make the problem worse. Antihistamines like diphenhydramine (Benadryl), diuretics like furosemide (Lasix), antinausea medications like prochlorperazine (Compazine), and many pain medicines can make your mouth dry. Your mouth can also become dry if you're not drinking enough fluids. Having a dry mouth can be uncomfortable, and it makes it hard for you to enjoy your food. Here are some suggestions to deal with this problem:

- Drink plenty of fluids—at least eight to ten glasses (eight ounces each) daily. Keep a water bottle handy as a reminder.

- Suck on ice chips; Popsicles; or tart, sugar-free candy.

- Chew sugar-free gum to increase your saliva.

- Moisten dry foods with liquids to make them easier to swallow. Add broth or warm milk to potatoes and gravy over meat or chicken.

- Use moisturizing lip balm for dry lips.

- Artificial saliva can be helpful. It's available without a prescription in the drugstore.

Mouth Soreness

During the months when you're receiving cancer treatments, there may be times when your mouth and throat become sore. The soreness may start with a feeling of hypersensitivity to sour or spicy tastes and some redness or swelling of your gums, cheeks, or throat. There may be open areas similar to cold sores on the sides of the inside of your mouth. Brushing your teeth, rinsing with a mouthwash, eating, or even swallowing may be painful.

Your doctor or nurse may call this condition *mucositis* or *stomatitis*. Mucositis means an inflammation of the mucous membranes of your digestive system, while stomatitis is an inflammation of the mucous linings of your mouth. Both terms describe the problems that may occur when the surface layer of cells lining your mouth and throat aren't replaced as quickly as usual because of the chemotherapy. If you have inflammation or soreness in your esophagus, it's called *esophagitis*.

Not everyone will develop mucositis, but it's good to be able to recognize the problem early and know what to do. While this condition can be painful and uncomfortable, but it will improve fairly quickly as the cells recuperate. When you experience mucositis, there are a number of things that can help you feel better, promote healing, and prevent infection.

SUGGESTIONS FOR MOUTH AND THROAT SORENESS

Keep your mouth clean and comfortable. First, the cleaner your mouth is, the better it will feel and the faster it will heal. Brushing your teeth or dentures and rinsing your mouth within thirty minutes after meals is very important.

When your mouth is sore or your platelet count is low, you need to be especially careful not to cause more irritation or bruising. Use a soft toothbrush. Wetting your toothbrush in hot water will soften the bristles even more. If your mouth is very sore, or your platelets are so low that gentle brushing causes bleeding, you can use a sponge-tipped swab to gently clean your mouth as well as to stimulate your mucous membranes. Although a sponge-tipped swab is not as effective as a toothbrush in removing debris or plaque from your teeth, it can help you get your teeth cleaner than just a rinse. Go back to using your toothbrush when your mouth tissues heal and your platelet count improves. If your platelet count is low, use the softest stream of water from a "water-jet" oral cleansing device to prevent bleeding.

Dentures and partials can cause some irritation to sensitive mouth tissues when these areas are sore, even if they fit well. It may help to remove them before sleeping at night or for short periods during the day. Try to keep your lips moist by using a lip gel or even a light layer of Vaseline. Most lip gels or balms have an oil base that will protect your lips for several hours. Some brands have sunscreen in them as well. Soon you'll notice that your dry lips are noticeably softer and that any cracks are beginning to heal.

If you have a sore mouth, avoid using commercial mouthwashes or products that contain alcohol or glycerin. Both will dry your mouth tissues even more and make the soreness worse. You can make a dilute solution of baking soda and warm water as a rinse. Use one half-teaspoon of baking soda mixed into a half-cup of water. The baking soda solution cleans, promotes healing, and lowers the acidity in your mouth. This is especially helpful if you've vomited and some of the stomach acid has come up into your mouth. Rinsing with a baking-soda solution will help to neutralize the effects of acidic debris on your tender oral tissues.

When your mouth or throat is sore, avoid hot or spicy foods. Foods that contain chili powder or pepper may cause more pain. Avoid drinks that are so hot that they make your mouth sting. Citrus juices (such as orange or grapefruit juices) and tomato juice may also be a problem, because they're acidic. Cool, bland fluids (apple juice, grape juice, pear nectar, herbal teas) will be more soothing to your mouth and throat.

Most people can cope with the short period when their mouths and throats are sore without too much difficulty. But if mouth pain is severe, it can interfere with your ability to eat or drink. When you have severe pain in other parts of your body, you would naturally try to protect that part by resting it until it no longer hurt. When your mouth hurts, however, that remedy isn't possible, since you must continue to take fluids and nourishment orally. So mouth pain that affects your ability to eat and drink should be reported to your doctor or nurse.

One thing your doctor can prescribe that may help is rinsing with a topical anesthetic (like the one the dentist uses before injections). This will temporarily relieve pain so that you can eat or clean your mouth. But be aware that if you swallow the numbing medicine, it will also suppress your natural gag reflex. Then you must be careful, because food or liquid can more easily be swallowed the "wrong way."

If your mouth pain is so severe that you can't eat or drink enough fluids to prevent dehydration, you may need to have IV fluids and pain medication for a few days until you feel better.

Taste Changes

After a time, some foods that previously tasted good to you may have a different, even unpleasant, flavor, or it may seem that flavors are diminished. For example, red meat may taste bitter, or sweet foods may taste more or less sweet than you're used to. Water may taste different—possibly metallic. The reason for this is that your taste buds may be temporarily altered by the way chemotherapy has affected the mucous membranes in your mouth. Even foods that you crave may taste different in an unpleasant way. Your sense of taste will eventually return to normal. But give it time; it may take several months after all your treatments are over. In the meantime, here are some things that may help.

Clean your mouth by brushing and rinsing with the baking-soda solution (described previously) before meals. When your mouth is clean and moist, flavors of foods may be more distinct. If your mouth feels stale, the taste of food won't be as pleasant.

Experiment with eating foods that have various kinds of flavors to see which ones taste good to you and which ones to avoid. When your sense of taste is diminished or altered, try eating foods with different textures or temperatures to make a meal more interesting.

If water tastes metallic, try filtering it with a filter pitcher or faucet attachment. Drinking flavored water may also help.

Chapter 7 ("Maintaining Good Nutrition") has more suggestions about how to deal with taste changes. A consultation with a nutritionist could help you find foods that are more appealing so that you can stay well nourished while experiencing this temporary problem.

Yeast Infection (Thrush)

There's a normal balance of organisms that naturally live in and on your body. When this balance changes, you're more likely to develop an infection. The normal balance of organisms that live in your mouth can change because of cancer treatments, medications, or a change in your nutrition.

White patches on the insides of your cheeks, on your tongue, or along the gum line may indicate that you have a yeast infection in your mouth (also known as *thrush*). Call your doctor or nurse to get a prescription for medication to eliminate the problem. There are two types of medications. One is a pill that you swallow called fluconazole (Diflucan). It works throughout your body to restore the normal level of flora. The second type of medicine comes in lozenge or liquid form (nystatin) and is applied directly in your mouth. Use the lozenges or liquid after eating, brushing, and rinsing, and don't rinse again for at least thirty minutes. In that way you can keep the medicine on the affected areas to promote healing.

If the medication comes as a lozenge, let it melt slowly in your mouth so that it can cover all your mouth surfaces as well as your throat. If you have difficulty with the lozenges because your mouth is very dry or sore, tell your doctor or nurse to order the medication in a liquid form.

When using the liquid, take about two teaspoons of it and swish it around in your mouth so that it covers all of the surfaces of your cheeks and gums. Then let it roll back into your throat and gargle with it so that it can also coat your throat. You can then either swallow it or spit it out. (Since your esophagus may also be sore or infected, swallowing the solution will allow it to coat and heal this area as well.)

Another way to take the solution is to measure out your doses into ice cube trays and freeze them. Then, when it's time to take your next dose of nystatin, you can pop a "nystatin-sicle" into your mouth. As it melts, it can provide soothing coolness and comfort to your tissues.

APPETITE PROBLEMS

Chemotherapy can temporarily affect your appetite. The medications you're taking may reduce your feelings of hunger so that you don't feel like eating much. Or they may change your appetite so that certain foods no longer appeal to you. Even though you know you need to maintain good nutrition at this time, it's hard to have an appetite if you're experiencing nausea, taste changes, constipation, fatigue, or pain. If you have any of these symptoms, relieving them can help improve your appetite.

Feeling full. Your digestive system may slow down at times during chemo so that your food takes longer to move through. When you feel that food is "sitting in your stomach," you may have a feeling of fullness or nausea, and eating anything else may be difficult. With or without nausea or the feeling of fullness, your appetite may wane while you're getting treatment. A large plate of food (even something you might like) can make you feel overwhelmed or discouraged. One way of coping with this feeling is to eat five or six small meals spaced throughout the day instead of three large meals.

Fatigue. If you're having problems with fatigue, just making a meal can be so exhausting that you lose the desire to eat. Some people cope with this problem by freezing single portions of homemade meals or buying frozen dinners. On days when you don't have the energy to cook, you can heat up a frozen meal with minimal effort.

Taste changes. If food seems tasteless, it's not as appetizing. Try eating foods with stronger flavors—spicy, sweet, or sour—so that they're more interesting. Stimulate your appetite with foods prepared and served attractively, perhaps shared with a friend. So much of our social and family interaction revolves around eating together. You may find that food tastes better when you eat with others.

Your doctor may prescribe medicine to stimulate your appetite or speed up the movement of food through your digestive system to help relieve the feeling of nausea or fullness. Your nutritionist may have other suggestions to help you maintain good nutrition until your appetite returns to normal.

Food Aversions

During this period of time when you may be experiencing nausea or taste changes, you may find that some foods seem particularly unappealing or even disgusting. This learned response is not unusual when you associate a particular food or taste with an unpleasant experience. For example, if you ate a tuna salad sandwich that caused food poisoning (hours of abdominal pain, nausea, and vomiting), you might not want to eat tuna salad again for a long time. This is an example of food aversion caused by an association with an unpleasant experience. It's not uncommon for people who experience uncontrolled nausea or other digestion problems to develop an aversion to something they ingested prior to that distress.

One way to avoid food aversions is to prevent nausea from developing or relieve it as soon as possible by taking the antinausea medications as prescribed. Another way to avoid developing food aversions when you feel nauseated is to eat a variety of different foods and flavors. Those foods should be bland and easily digested, and leave no lingering taste or smell. That way, you don't associate one particular food or flavor with the unpleasant feeling. Some examples are applesauce, mashed potatoes, rice, yogurt, and cottage cheese.

Sometimes, in an attempt to stimulate your appetite, a family member will prepare your "favorite" food after chemotherapy. They may be surprised and disappointed that after a while you can no longer stand the sight or smell of that old favorite.

HEARTBURN

The glands of the stomach contain cells that secrete gastric juices to aid in digestion. One of the components of gastric juices is hydrochloric acid. Certain chemicals, such as *histamine*, stimulate the secretion of hydrochloric acid into the stomach. When histamine attaches to sites on the cells called H2 receptors, it signals the cells to secrete stomach acid. These gastric cells also have acid-producing systems called *proton pumps*, which produce acid and release it into the stomach.

Heartburn (also called acid indigestion or gastric reflux) is a burning sensation in the stomach, chest, or throat. It happens when stomach acid irritates your esophagus. If the muscular valve between the esophagus and stomach doesn't close well, stomach acid can back up (reflux) into the esophagus and cause irritation.

Reflux usually occurs just after eating or if you lie down while your stomach is full. If you need to lie down, keep your upper body elevated with a pillow or cushion. Smoking aggravates heartburn, because it increases the production of acid and relaxes the valve between your stomach and esophagus. Certain foods, such as caffeinated beverages, alcohol, chocolate, tomatoes, onions, garlic, and citrus fruits, will also relax the valve and contribute to heartburn.

If chemotherapy has made the lining of your stomach more sensitive to the acid, you may need to take medication to neutralize or turn off the acid production in your stomach.

Medications to Relieve Heartburn

Antacids neutralize the acid already in your stomach, thereby reducing the irritation in that area. They can provide quick relief of symptoms for a short period of time. Examples of common antacids are TUMS, Maalox, Mylanta, and Rolaids. Antacids are available without a prescription.

H2 blockers reduce the production of acid in your stomach. They do this by blocking the chemical histamine from stimulating the acid-producing cells lining the stomach. H2 blockers don't relieve symptoms as fast as antacids, but they can relieve symptoms for a longer period of time. Some examples are cimetidine (Tagamet), famotidine (Pepcid), and ranitidine (Zantac). Most H2 blockers are available without a prescription.

If antacids or H2 blockers don't relieve your heartburn symptoms, your doctor may prescribe a *proton pump inhibitor*. These reduce stomach-acid production by inhibiting the enzyme pump process so that acid isn't produced and released into the stomach. Examples are omeprazole (Prilosec), lansopraxole (Prevacid), pantoprozole

(Protonix), rabeprazole (Aciphex), and esomeprazole (Nexium). These drugs can take up to four days to work but can be very effective for relieving symptoms. Some proton pump inhibitors are available without a prescription.

Be sure to let your physician know if you're experiencing heartburn, when it occurs, and what nonprescription medicines you're taking for relief. This information will help your physician determine the treatment most likely to relieve your symptoms.

DIARRHEA

When you have diarrhea, food moves through your large intestine so quickly that the water can't be absorbed normally. Therefore, your bowel movements are more liquid and more frequent. This problem can be very distressing and disruptive to your normal activities as well as severe fluid loss and imbalances in the salts and minerals your body needs. There are a number of different reasons why people getting chemotherapy can develop diarrhea.

Effects of cancer treatments. Chemotherapy can damage the cells in the intestinal tract that divide frequently. That can make the rhythmic movement of your intestines (peristalsis) speed up, and anything in the intestine moves out rapidly in the form of liquid stools. Diarrhea will usually abate when the intestinal lining heals.

Effects of medications. Metoclopramide (Reglan), which can be used for nausea, increases the movement of food and fluid through the digestive tract. This may relieve the feeling of stomach fullness after eating, but it can sometimes cause loose stools.

Effects of infection. Diarrhea can also be caused by infection. Since chemotherapy suppresses your immune system, you have fewer white blood cells to fight infection. As a result, bacteria that normally live within your digestive system can cause infections when your defenses are temporarily weakened by the treatments.

What to Do When You Have Diarrhea

If you have frequent loose stools, call your doctor or nurse right away. Be ready to describe:

- the frequency and approximate amount of your stools

- your weight (weigh yourself before you call)

- the amounts and types of fluids you're drinking

When you have diarrhea, you can lose so much fluid that you become dehydrated. Along with the fluid, you also lose important minerals (especially potassium). If severe diarrhea goes untreated, you may experience other signs of dehydration, such as feeling dizzy or weak. Your kidneys will make less urine in an attempt to hold onto fluid, and therefore they can't remove waste products adequately.

For all of these reasons, it's important to keep drinking lots of fluids and replacing lost minerals. Try slowly sipping small amounts of fluids such as fruit juices and nectars, soups, and sports drinks formulated to replace lost electrolytes. Since drinking very cold fluids can irritate your intestines and cause more discomfort, try drinking moderately cool or lukewarm fluids. If you feel like drinking sodas such as ginger ale, it's best to let the "fizz" out first so that you won't feel bloated. (The carbonation in the soda can also irritate your throat as it goes down.)

While you have diarrhea, avoid foods that can make it worse, such as dairy products, greasy fried foods, caffeinated beverages, and chocolate. Bland, easily digested foods, such as bananas, apple-sauce, rice, toast, crackers, and broth, are less likely to stimulate more diarrhea.

Infection

Diarrhea can be your body's way of getting rid of the organism causing an infection or the toxic products produced by the organism, so you may be asked to collect a small amount of stool so that it can be tested for infection.

If the stool sample shows that you have an infection, you'll first be given an antibiotic to start eliminating the infection, and then medication to slow down the diarrhea. Loperamide (Imodium) or diphenoxylate and atropine (Lomotil) will slow down the rhythmic movement of your intestine and allow liquid to be absorbed from the stool, producing firmer bowel movements.

CONSTIPATION

Constipation is a decrease in the usual frequency of bowel movements. When you're constipated, the stool stays in your intestines longer, so it may become very dry and hard. There are a number of reasons why you could become constipated during this time. Anything that slows the movement of your intestines will cause constipation, and some chemotherapy drugs such as Vincristine (Oncovin, Vincasar) cause your intestines to slow down. You can become constipated if you're taking pain medicines frequently, because they, too, will slow the digestive tract. Also, some antinausea drugs like granisetron (Kytril) and ondansetron (Zofran) can be constipating. If you're less active than usual, the normal rhythm of your intestines is slowed. If you're not eating or drinking as much as you usually do because of nausea, fatigue, or a poor appetite, you can become dehydrated, leading to constipation.

What to Do to Prevent Constipation

If you're at risk for constipation due to one of the reasons above, it's a good idea to follow these suggestions to prevent it from happening and making you uncomfortable.

Increase fluids. Just increasing the amount of fluids you drink will help your bowel movements become softer. Warm, noncaffeinated liquids such as herbal teas, fruit juices, and prune juice will help keep your intestines moving and prevent constipation.

Eat high-fiber foods. Foods such as raw vegetables, beans, fresh and dried fruits, and high-fiber cereals increase the bulk in your stools and stimulate the intestines to move. But if you increase the fiber in your diet, be sure to increase the fluids you drink. If you increase the bulk without increasing the fluid, you'll become more constipated than before.

Increase activity. There are a number of reasons why you may be less active. Your usual routines might be changed drastically because of the necessity of keeping appointments at the clinic, hospital, lab, or doctor's office. Besides, you may just feel a lot more fatigued than usual during this time. Pain medications or antinausea medications may also make you sleepy and less active. Or, you may have less energy because you aren't eating or sleeping as well. But even if you're not up to your usual exercise program, some activity may help relieve constipation. Just taking a short walk each day in the fresh air will make a difference.

Medications to Relieve Constipation

If you haven't had a bowel movement in two or more days, you may need a laxative, a stool softener, or an enema. Although many of these remedies are available without a prescription, check with your doctor before taking any to make sure that you use the right one for you.

Stool softeners work by combining or mixing with the stool to make it oilier or more liquid. Colace, docusate sodium, and DSS are examples of stool softeners. Oil-based suppositories such as glycerin work in much the same way.

Laxatives stimulate the intestines to move the stool along at a faster rate and thus prevent the stool from getting too hard or dry. Drugs such as senna, castor oil, cascara, and Ducolax increase the movement in the intestines by irritation. The intestines moves faster in an attempt to remove the irritating substance from the body sooner.

Bulk-forming laxatives such as Metamucil and Citrucel contain indigestible products such as bran and methylcellulose, which increase the volume of the stool in your intestines. When your stool has more bulk, the feeling of fullness in your rectum stimulates the urge to have a bowel movement. Fruits and vegetables work the same way, because the indigestible portions of those foods contribute to the bulk of your stool. Fiber supplements must be taken with adequate fluids, because fiber without fluid becomes hard and difficult to pass.

Milk of magnesia contains nonabsorbable salts, which help retain fluid in your stool. With the increase in fluid, the stool is bulkier and thus stimulates the urge to have a bowel movement. Miralax brings water into the bowel, making the stool softer and easier to pass.

Enemas work to stimulate your lower intestine by irritation or by increasing the volume of the colon contents. That stimulates the colon to contract. Be sure to check with your doctor before using an enema or any medication rectally. When your white-blood-cell count or platelet count is low, there's a greater chance of bleeding or infection.

IN CONCLUSION

There are many products that are effective in relieving digestion problems. Some of these products are now available without a prescription. You probably have a medicine cabinet full of remedies, with everything from antacids to suppositories. But when you're getting chemotherapy, talk with your doctor or nurse to be sure that what you're taking will be safe and effective for you.

Chapter 7

Maintaining Good Nutrition
By Tinrin Chew, RD, CSO

Food is the fuel of life. It's the raw material that runs the machinery of your body. Good nutrition is important throughout your life, but it's even more crucial when you're preparing to embark on cancer-fighting treatments. It's important that you maintain your body weight and lean-muscle mass. You need to rebuild healthy cells, repair tissues, fight infection, and recover from the effects of chemotherapy. Good nutrition can also improve your sense of well-being and even increase the potential for a favorable response to treatment.

Of course, food also provides more than fuel. It's a way to nurture yourself and to socialize with family and friends. Preparing and serving food is a way many people show their love and concern for others. During treatment, when your appetite or sense of taste changes (even temporarily), it can also affect how you enjoy and share this part of your life.

GETTING READY

Before starting any cancer-fighting treatment, many people may already be experiencing nutritional deficiencies or unintentional weight loss. This can happen because cancer cells are rapidly growing and dividing, and they use the vitamins, minerals, proteins, and calories that the rest of your body needs. You may also be experiencing difficulty chewing, swallowing, or digesting your food. While you're recovering from the effects of surgery, you may be taking antibiotics or pain medicines. These drugs can also affect your appetite, digestion, energy, and ability to taste or enjoy your food as you normally do.

Many people are tempted to try a radical diet change or start taking multiple herbal and dietary supplements. However, during this stressful time of your life, you may not be able to make many dietary changes, despite how good they may sound. Don't feel pressured to make changes now; you can do it gradually as you feel better or after your treatment is completed.

Your immediate goal is to eat and drink well enough to get through your chemotherapy with minimal problems. When you're done with treatment, consider further dietary and lifestyle modification for the long haul—survivorship and thriving.

A consultation with a nutritionist before starting treatment is a great way to get information about the food (fuel) your body needs to renew, rebuild, recover, get strong, and get ready.

WEIGHT GAIN AND WEIGHT LOSS

Once you start treatment, it's best to keep your weight as stable as possible. This is not the time to lose unwanted pounds. Numerous studies have shown that unintentional weight loss during treatment can compromise your immune function and your ability to recover from the effects of chemotherapy. Thus, it's better to lose weight after you've recovered from your cancer treatment. On the other hand, some people actually gain weight during chemotherapy. This may be due to medications, changes in their eating habits, or less physical activity. However, studies have shown that too much weight gain during treatment can also adversely affect you. The goal is to not lose or gain more than 5 percent of your weight throughout your treatment.

CHEMO CYCLES

The way chemotherapy affects your appetite or digestion varies depending on the kind of chemotherapy you receive. It also varies at different times during your treatment. Chemotherapy is given in *cycles*. The period of time between one treatment and the next is considered to be a cycle. The *chemo phase* of the cycle is the first few days after your chemotherapy. The *rebuilding phase* is the rest of the time until you receive treatment again. Nausea, constipation, or fatigue may be a problem during the chemo phase. Diarrhea or mouth soreness may be a problem a week or so later, during the rebuilding phase. Because your symptoms may change over time, you also need to change how you eat so you can stay well nourished during both phases.

Good Nutrition for the Chemo Phase

The antinausea medications available now are much better at preventing and relieving the nausea caused by chemotherapy than the medications used years ago. But during the first few days after chemotherapy, you could still feel somewhat queasy. The smell of food may bother you, and you may experience changes in taste. Your first line of defense is the nausea-blocking and nausea-relieving medicines. You should take them as directed by your doctor and nurse.

They'll also tell you to "push fluids" in order to flush out the chemotherapy by-products and waste products from your system. This will protect your kidneys (your body's filtering system) and help you feel better. But what should you drink? And how much? What should you eat? Here are some guidelines.

FLUID GUIDELINES FOR THE CHEMO PHASE

A simple rule to follow is to take your weight (in pounds) and divide by two. That's the number of ounces you should drink each day. One cup of fluid is eight ounces. So, for example, a person weighing 160 pounds (160 divided by 2 is 80) should try to drink 80 ounces or 10 cups of fluids per day. This is especially important for the first three to four days after treatment. (If you're significantly overweight, your nutritionist or physician can help you calculate the amount of fluids you should drink.)

"Pushing fluids" doesn't mean to just drink water or sports beverages. Many chemotherapy drugs can deplete important elements within your body (such as sodium and potassium). If you don't replace them, in a few days you could feel worse instead of better. That's why it's important to drink the right amounts and the right types of fluids. The following chart shows a balance of different kinds of fluids.

Fluid Guidelines Chart

25% (sodium)	25% (water)
Broth	Water
Miso soup	Weak tea or herbal tea
Chicken rice soup	
Chicken noodle soup	
25% (whatever you like)	25% (potassium)
Watermelon	Apricot nectar
Popsicle	Peach nectar
Sherbet	Prune juice
Jell-O	Apple juice
Ginger ale	Grape juice
Gatorade or sports drink	Milk
Pedialyte	Yogurt smoothie

Many people find that watermelon is great after chemo. It's high in fluid content and potassium, and provides calories when you may not feel like eating solid food. By sprinkling it with salt, you help meet your sodium needs. Think of it as killing four birds with one stone: fluid, calories, potassium, and sodium in one food.

Space out your fluid intake throughout the day. Don't try to drink a large amount of fluids at one time. If you do, you could feel overfull afterward, and that can contribute to feeling nauseated.

Alcohol should not be consumed during this phase.

FOOD GUIDELINES FOR THE CHEMO PHASE

Right after your treatment, you may feel fine and want to eat a large meal. Resist the urge to do that, especially if this is your first treatment and you don't know how you'll feel later. The antinausea medications may protect you from nausea initially, but you may not digest or empty your stomach as you normally do. You could end up feeling bloated and nauseated after a large, heavy meal.

During the chemo phase, many people find that eating smaller portions more frequently, instead of three large meals, is better. Try to eat something every three hours. Eat bland, low-fat, and low-acidity foods. Also, eat foods that have less odor.

Some people who feel slightly nauseated or queasy may eat very little or nothing at all, because they're afraid of feeling worse or vomiting. But when your stomach is empty, you can experience stomach pain, and that can make you feel even more nauseated. It's a good idea to eat dry, starchy foods to calm mild nausea and soak up acid in your stomach. Examples of starchy foods are potatoes, saltine crackers, bagels, bread, and plain bean-and-rice burritos.

Some people wake up feeling nauseated on an empty stomach. They may have a hard time keeping anything down—even pills. If this happens to you, try to focus your eyes and breathe slowly and evenly for a few minutes. After a few breaths, start eating a few bites of dry, starchy foods (like crackers) and continue to breathe slowly and evenly. In a few minutes, you'll feel better, and then you can take your antinausea medication.

Greasy and spicy foods are not only poorly tolerated but may also give off a lot of odor. Colder foods, room-temperature foods, and foods with little or no odor are usually better tolerated. Eating in a relaxed environment with good ventilation helps decrease nausea and improve your appetite. You may also find that acidic foods upset your stomach. Acidic foods include tomatoes, tomato sauces, oranges, and orange juice.

Try *not* to eat your favorite food during this time. If you happen to feel nauseated because of the chemotherapy, you don't want to associate this uncomfortable feeling with the food you just ate. Avoiding your favorite foods now will help prevent their becoming unappealing later.

SAMPLE MENU FOR THE CHEMO PHASE

The following is a sample menu of small meals and snacks that are nutritional and well tolerated during this phase.

Breakfast: Toast and jelly, poached egg, tea

Snack: Cottage cheese and cantaloupe, grape juice

Lunch: Chicken-rice soup, turkey sandwich with light mayonnaise, tea

Snack: Watermelon

Dinner: Roasted chicken, baked potato with a small amount of butter, green beans

Snack: Yogurt and saltine crackers

OTHER SUGGESTIONS FOR THE CHEMO PHASE

If you're unable to eat much the first few days after chemo, don't worry. Your goal is to drink plenty of fluids and eat what you can tolerate. But if you're unable to drink adequately or eat any solid food, be sure to call your doctor's office. Don't wait until you get dehydrated. You may need extra IV fluids and more or a different nausea-relieving medicine to help you feel better so that you can resume eating and drinking on your own.

Here are several other suggestions that can help at this time:

- Brushing your teeth and rinsing your mouth can help your appetite by getting rid of a sour taste that can interfere with your enjoyment of food.

- Constipation can make you feel bloated or nauseated and can interfere with eating and drinking adequately. Many nausea-blocking medicines as well as many pain medicines can cause this problem. Ask your doctor if and when you should take a stool softener or laxative to prevent or relieve constipation.

- Although some chemotherapy drugs can cause diarrhea immediately after treatment, most diarrhea, if it occurs, happens about a week after treatment. Therefore if you're regularly using a laxative, be cautious for about five or six days after your chemotherapy. (Chapter 6, "Coping with Other Digestion Changes," has additional information about preventing and managing both diarrhea and constipation.)

- Stay active without getting overly tired. Studies have repeatedly shown the benefits of exercise during chemotherapy. Physical activity during the chemo phase increases circulation, helps your body clear toxins, relieves nausea, increases appetite, and helps you feel better.

SUPPLEMENT AND VITAMIN GUIDELINES FOR THE CHEMO PHASE

Unless specifically prescribed by your doctor or nutritionist, it's safer not to take any supplements or vitamins during the chemo phase (the day of treatment and for three to four days after). Your body is working very hard to eliminate toxins. Many vitamins and supplements add an extra burden for the liver to process without much benefit. There are a few specific supplements, such as glutamine, that are useful during this phase to decrease some chemotherapy-related side effects. Talk to your doctor or nutritionist to get advice about what supplements you can take at this time.

Good Nutrition for the Rebuilding Phase

Once the chemo phase is over, you'll probably begin to feel better. This is when your body is working to rebuild so that you'll be ready for the next cycle of chemo. If you have lost a pound or two during the first few days after chemo, you should gain it back during this time. Two or three meals a day may not be enough for you to regain weight, especially if your appetite is poor. So try adding two or three snacks in addition to meals. You may try snacks such as yogurt, protein bars or energy bars, avocado, nuts and seeds, trail mix, nut butters and crackers, hard-boiled eggs, pudding, cottage cheese and fruit, and single-serving-sized canned fruit, tuna, or chicken.

FLUID GUIDELINES FOR THE REBUILDING PHASE

Keep up your fluid intake. It's not as important to drink soups or fruit juices (which replace electrolytes, such as sodium and potassium) unless you're experiencing diarrhea. If you feel well and have a good appetite, you should focus on drinking sugar-free beverages, such as decaf or herbal tea, water, and vegetable juices. If you find that you have difficulty eating solid food and are losing weight, it certainly is a good idea to drink nutrient- and calorie-dense beverages, such as fruit and yogurt smoothies; protein shakes; soups; and other nutritional beverages, such as Carnation Instant Breakfast, Ensure, Boost, Resurgex, and Resource Support. Look for supplements that are fortified with vitamins and minerals and have at least 10 grams of protein and 200 calories per serving. It's also beneficial to choose a product that contains 2 to 4 grams of fiber per serving. If you have diabetes, look for products designed for diabetics.

FOOD GUIDELINES FOR THE REBUILDING PHASE

Eating a balance of protein, fruits, vegetables, whole grains, and healthy fats at this time will help your body to repair, rebuild, and gain back any weight you've lost.

Protein. During the rebuilding phase, it's important to take in enough protein to help build cells. Think of protein as the bricks that you need to build a strong house. Every time you eat, try to include some kind of protein. Good protein foods include fish, chicken, lean meats, eggs, and cottage cheese. Whole grains and beans eaten together, such as rice and beans or whole-wheat tortillas and beans, are also good sources of protein. Whey protein powder is another source. You could add a tablespoon or two of protein powder to cooked cereal, gravy, or smoothies. Keep a protein bar or energy bar in your bag. You can munch on it anytime.

Fruits, vegetables, and grains. They're important too. Try to eat at least five to seven servings of fruits and vegetables each day during the rebuilding phase. They contain *phytochemicals* (or *phytonutrients*). These are compounds found in plants that can protect healthy cells, regulate cancer-cell growth, modulate hormone balance, and block carcinogen formation or neutralize their impact on healthy cells. Phytochemicals also act as powerful antioxidants to protect healthy cells and newly generated cells. Eating fruits, vegetables, and whole grains gives you greater benefits than taking a single vitamin pill.

Cooked vegetables are usually better tolerated than raw vegetables, especially when you're experiencing digestive difficulties such as loose bowels or heartburn. Good vegetable choices during this time include all the winter and summer squashes; carrots; green beans; asparagus; peas; beets; and tender, leafy greens.

Cooked fruits are usually better tolerated than raw fruits, and peeled fruits are better tolerated than fruits with skin on. You may enjoy papaya, pears, bananas, melons, apples, and avocados, because these are more easily digested during this time.

Whole grains are important, too. To get enough whole grains, start the day with a bowl of oatmeal. Then eat two to three servings of whole grains, beans, or peas later in the day.

If your mouth is sore or if you have indigestion or diarrhea, you may find it difficult to eat enough fruits, vegetables, and whole grains. You might find that creamed or pureed vegetable soups, such as butternut-squash soup and ginger-carrot soup, taste good and are more easily digested. Smoothies made with yogurt and fruit also contain phytochemicals, taste good, and are well tolerated.

Fats and oils. Fats and oils give you the most calories. If you're losing weight, use them liberally. However, if you're gaining weight, use them sparingly. Some oils are better for you than others.

Good oils and fats include olive oil, canola oil, avocados, flaxseed oil, nuts, and oil from fish. These oils are either monounsaturated fats or contain high amounts of omega-3 fats. They have anti-inflammatory effects and many health benefits. Use these oils for good health and to gain weight. Avocado is a wonderful high-fat snack. Remember to keep flaxseed oil in the refrigerator, because it's not as stable as other types of oil, and it shouldn't be cooked. (It's great in a salad dressing.)

Other fats and oils, such as regular margarine, hydrogenated vegetable oils, corn oil, and other vegetable or seed oils are high in saturated fats, trans fats, or omega-6 fats. These fats promote inflammation in the body and decrease immune function. Avoid these fats and oils as much as possible. These fats are also found in many baked goods, dessert items, fried foods, convenience foods, and processed foods.

Years ago your nutritionist might have suggested that you add extra calories by eating lots of ice cream, cheese, butter, margarine, cream, sour cream, cream cheese, or cookies and cakes. But studies have shown that the excessive intake of fats and sweets drives up the inflammatory process and isn't good for your immune function or overall health. Cake and cookies, ice cream, and other treats can be comfort foods, and you can enjoy them occasionally. But in general, avoid eating high-fat, empty-calorie foods.

SUPPLEMENTS AND FUNCTIONAL FOODS FOR THE REBUILDING PHASE

It's always a good idea to let your doctor know the nutritional supplements you're taking or intend to take during your chemotherapy. There might be some that you should not take because of the kind of cancer you have, the kind of chemotherapy you're receiving, other medications you're taking, or some other preexisting condition you have. Bring in your supplements and review them with your doctor and the nutritionist in your clinic.

Daily multiple-vitamin and mineral supplements. Even if you're eating a good, balanced diet, nutrient absorption can be significantly decreased by digestive difficulties, chemotherapy, and many medications. So taking a daily vitamin and mineral supplement is a good idea to meet your body's increased needs while you're going through the rebuilding phase.

Probiotics. Normally, there are many microorganisms lining your gut that aid in digestion and nutrient absorption. These microorganisms are called *probiotics*; they're the opposite of antibiotics. When you take probiotics, you get the benefit of these "friendly" organisms. Lactobacillus and bifidobacterium are the most widely used probiotic bacteria. They're found in fermented foods, such as yogurt, kefir, miso, and tempeh.

You can also take probiotic supplements. Some require refrigeration and some don't, so check the label carefully. Also, look for a product that has more than two strains of bacteria and at least ten billion live bacteria. It's particularly important to replace these useful microorganisms after a course of antibiotics. Those medicines kill off the "good bacteria" along with the bad bacteria that caused your infection, and that can lead to diarrhea. Replacing the microorganisms by taking probiotics can lessen the problem.

Probiotics are also helpful in improving immune function, decreasing gut infection, and reducing inflammation of the bowel. They can also help your digestion if you have milk or lactose intolerance, and they can possibly prevent yeast infection. Eating a cup of yogurt daily would be a way to keep good bacteria working for you.

Prebiotics. These are nondigestible food substances, such as fiber, that stimulate the growth and activity of beneficial microorganisms already in your colon. Therefore, they work together with probiotics to keep your gut healthy. Dietary sources of prebiotics include soybeans, whole grains, bananas, onions, garlic, leeks, and Jerusalem artichokes. You can also take prebiotic supplements, such as inulin and FOS. Many probiotic supplements may already contain inulin or FOS.

Eating hint. A cup of low-fat organic plain yogurt over banana and berries topped with a spoonful of ground flaxmeal provides your body with a combination of probiotics, prebiotics, and omega-3 fats.

Glutamine. Proteins are made up of amino acids. Glutamine is an amino acid that has been shown to improve the mucous membrane lining of the digestive system. So this supplement can be helpful for people getting chemo who have mouth soreness or diarrhea. Glutamine may help repair the mucous membrane of your entire digestive tract and reduce these side effects. You could mix one to two teaspoons of glutamine with water, rinse your mouth, and swallow. Doing this three times a day can promote healing and reduce pain.

Certain chemotherapy drugs can cause numbness and tingling sensations at your fingertips, your toes, or the bottoms of your feet. This is called *peripheral neuropathy*. Glutamine seems to reduce these symptoms as well.

Omega-3 fish oil. Fatty fish and fish oils contain *eicosapentaenoic acid* (*EPA*) and *docosahexaenoic acid* (*DHA*), which have been shown to reduce inflammation and the growth rate of tumors. Animal studies also suggest that they can increase the effectiveness of chemotherapy in killing tumor cells. Recent research has also shown that taking two grams of EPA daily can help stop weight loss and muscle loss caused by cancer and can possibly help improve appetite. Eating fish two to three times a week is a good way to get omega-3 fats. Or you can take a fish-oil supplement. Start slowly, taking one teaspoon of fish oil liquid or two fish-oil capsules a day.

SAMPLE MENU FOR THE REBUILDING PHASE

Here's a sample menu with healthy, balanced foods that can help your body repair and rebuild so that you're ready for your next chemo cycle.

Breakfast:

Oatmeal with blueberries, sprinkled with cinnamon (if you need extra calories, mix some flaxseed oil into oatmeal)

Two poached eggs (if you don't want eggs, add one scoop of protein powder to oatmeal)

Hot tea or hot cocoa

Lunch:

Butternut-squash soup

Turkey sandwich on whole-grain bread (with avocado, tomato, and light mayonnaise)

Fresh fruit

Snack:

Homemade trail mix (walnuts, raisins, and pretzel sticks)

Pomegranate juice (1/2 cup with 3/4 cup water or sparkling water) or vegetable juice

Dinner:

Baked salmon

Steamed vegetables (try at least two vegetables, such as asparagus and red bell pepper) drizzled with olive oil

Rice

A piece of dark chocolate

Herbal tea

Snack:

Low-fat plain yogurt over fruit (sprinkle yogurt with one tablespoon ground flax meal or wheat germ)

Drink water or tea throughout the day

RECOMMENDATIONS FOR DIGESTIVE DIFFICULTIES

Chemo can cause a variety of side effects that can affect the digestive system. These side effects can affect your ability to eat and drink adequately and absorb nutrients.

However, there are many things you can do to manage these side effects.

Nausea

Nausea medications can be very effective for preventing or relieving nausea from chemo. However, some people may still have some queasy feelings or nausea. If you're taking the medications prescribed by your doctor but still feel nauseated or if you have any vomiting, call your doctor or nurse to get an evaluation. The following recommendations can also help prevent or relieve nausea:

- Eat small amounts and eat often. Eat every two to three hours.

- Eat and drink slowly.

- Eat dry foods, such as saltines, pretzels, bagels, toast, and baked potatoes.

- Eat cold or room-temperature foods, such as sandwiches, cottage cheese and fruit, and hard-boiled eggs. Hot foods produce odors that may add to the nausea.

- Drink only small amounts of liquids with meals. Drinking large amounts of liquids can cause a full, bloated feeling.

- Drink cool or chilled beverages. Sip liquids throughout the day.

- Eat foods that are bland (not spicy) and low fat.

- Rest after meals. It's best to rest sitting up or with your head elevated at least four inches for about an hour after meals.

- Try peppermint or ginger tea; it may reduce nausea.

- Limit unpleasant odors, sights, and sounds; they may aggravate nausea.

- Keep your room well ventilated. Avoid rooms that are stuffy or too warm, or have cooking odors.

- If taste changes occur, suck on sugar-free hard candy such as peppermints, sour balls, or lemon drops.

- Avoid too much activity and sudden movements that may interfere with your sense of balance. Dizziness can make you feel more nauseated.

- Rinse your mouth frequently to avoid unpleasant tastes.

- Learn relaxation techniques that involve deep rhythmic breathing and quiet concentration. This can be helpful before, during, and after meals.

Taste Changes

This is a common experience after getting chemotherapy. It can last for a few days after your treatment or persist longer. Here are some suggestions to deal with this side effect:

- Rinse your mouth frequently to avoid unpleasant tastes.

- If you have a "metallic" taste in your mouth, use plastic utensils instead of regular silverware and avoid canned foods. Red meats contain more iron and other minerals. Thus, they may taste more metallic than eggs and cheese. Temporarily avoid the offensive foods and substitute other high-protein foods, such as eggs, milk, cheese, tofu, beans, and rice.

- Try flavoring your food with different or unusual flavors, such as sweet and sour, citrus, lemon zest, mustard wine sauces, tomato or fruit salsa, and different spices. If your sense of taste is dulled, you may find that foods with strong flavors taste better.

- Try to eat cold foods that don't have much odor. Yogurts, cottage cheese with fruit, smoothies, and shakes are all good choices.

- If food tastes too sweet, try adding salt to it. Adding sour or tart to fruit smoothies can decrease sweetness. Don't do this if you have a sore mouth or throat. Adding a teaspoon of instant coffee to a chocolate or vanilla shake, or liquid nutrition beverage such as Ensure, can reduce the sweet taste.

If your appetite is affected because food tastes differently, talk with your doctor about trying a short course of a zinc supplement. This may help you to regain your sense of taste.

Sore Mouth and Throat

Some chemo drugs are more likely to cause mouth and throat soreness. These suggestions can help improve your comfort if this happens to you:

- Keep your mouth clean by rinsing after meals, snacks, or fruit juices. Follow mouth-care directions given by your doctor or nurse.

- Eat soft, moist foods that are cool or room temperature. Canned fruits, yogurt, poached eggs, egg salad, pudding, bread soaked with milk, pureed or blenderized vegetable soups and fruits, mashed potatoes, and thin cooked cereals are easier to eat.

- Stay away from spicy, hot, salty, or acidic foods. Food made with tomatoes, tomato sauce, citrus, or other fruit juices can be irritating.

- Use a straw to drink liquids to bypass sore areas in the mouth.

- Try sucking on ice or frozen fruit, such as frozen grapes or watermelon.

- Extra gravy and sauces can help you swallow more easily if your throat is sore.

- Try glutamine (5 grams) mixed with about 3/4 cup of water. Rinse, gargle, and hold it in your mouth for about thirty seconds; then swallow. Do this three times a day to speed up healing of your mouth and throat.

Constipation

You may experience constipation the first few days after chemotherapy. Some nausea-blocking medicines and pain medicines can cause this problem. Your doctor may have prescribed a stool softener or a laxative to help you move your bowels. Here are more suggestions:

- Drink at least eight to ten cups of fluids daily. Warm fluids may be especially helpful. Try a cup of warm prune juice or a laxative tea.

- Slowly add more fiber to your diet, such as fresh fruits, dried fruits, nuts, vegetables, beans, and high-fiber cereals.

- Eat a good breakfast. Include a hot drink and high-fiber foods, either bran cereals or whole-grain toast.

- Try to be more active.

Diarrhea

Diarrhea is a serious problem, because you lose both fluid and important electrolytes that your body needs. So if you have loose, watery stools; blood in your stools; a fever; or a tender and bloated abdomen, be sure to check with your doctor. You may need lab tests, IV fluids, or antibiotics to control and resolve this problem. It's important to take action right away when you have frequent watery or loose stools. Uncontrolled diarrhea can lead to dehydration, weakness, and poor nutrient absorption.

What you choose to eat or drink can make a big difference in controlling or preventing diarrhea. Here are some recommendations:

- Be sure to drink plenty of fluids to prevent dehydration.

- Be sure to sip a variety of fluids, such as broth, electrolyte drinks such as Pedialyte, diluted fruit juices, and nectars. Sip liquid slowly but constantly, all day.

- After each loose bowel movement, add one additional cup of liquid.

- Eat small, frequent snacks or meals. Eating too much food at one time can overload your digestive tract and worsen diarrhea.

- Drink most liquids between meals. Drinking too much during a meal can overload your digestive system and result in diarrhea.

- Eat low-fat, plain yogurt daily. Yogurt contains probiotics. It may help you digest food better and restore some good bacteria to your digestive tract.

- Eat foods that are high in soluble fiber. These include oatmeal, bananas, applesauce, canned fruits, rice, pasta, potatoes without skin, white bread, and rice cereal. Soluble fibers help bulk up loose stool.

- Avoid foods that are high in insoluble fiber. These include fresh fruits with skin or peel, whole-wheat bread, pasta, raw vegetables, seeds, nuts, and popcorn. Insoluble fiber can worsen diarrhea.

- Avoid milk and food made with milk, or use lactose-free milk instead. Most people can tolerate yogurt.

- Avoid drinking alcohol and caffeinated beverages, such as coffee and tea, which can worsen diarrhea. Decaffeinated and herbal teas are okay.

- Avoid fatty or greasy foods, such as french fries, fried meats, bacon, pizza, rich desserts, doughnuts, pastries, potato chips, gravies, and high-fat dressings.

- Glutamine may help decrease diarrhea, because it helps rebuild the lining of the digestive tract. Mix 5 to 10 grams of glutamine with applesauce or diluted fruit juice or yogurt. Do this three times a day until diarrhea stops; then continue for a few more days. If the chemotherapy you receive is known to cause diarrhea, you can start using glutamine before it develops, as a preventative strategy.

Here are a few recipes to try if you're experiencing diarrhea.

Rice Congee: Combine one cup of uncooked rice with six to seven cups of water and one teaspoon of salt. Cook 45 minutes or until rice almost falls apart. Slowly eat the rice and sip the rice fluid.

Clove Tea: Combine six to eight cloves and one tea bag of herbal, noncaffeinated tea (try ginger or chamomile) in one cup of water. Simmer this mixture until the volume is reduced by half (until only 1/2 cup remains). Let cool until just warm, and drink.

World Health Organization (WHO) Rehydration Solution: Mix the following ingredients together:

1 cup orange juice (substitute noncitrus juice if your mouth is sore)

8 teaspoons sugar

3/4 teaspoon baking soda

1/2 teaspoon salt

1 liter water

Poor Appetite

If you find that you don't have much of an appetite, particularly during the rebuilding phase of your chemo cycle, follow these recommendations to increase the amount of food you can eat:

- Plan to eat five to six times a day. Don't wait to feel hungry. When you plan to eat at a set time, you're less likely to forget to eat or skip meals. Don't worry about how much; just focus on eating something.

- Have snack food handy. Keep some yogurt; cheese; hard-boiled eggs; single servings of soups, tuna, and canned fruit; energy bars; dried fruits; and nuts on hand.

- Cut up energy bars or protein bars into bite-sized pieces. Keep some dried fruits and nuts in your purse or pocket. You can eat a bite or two whenever you think of it.

- Focus on high-protein, high-calorie foods, such as peanut butter, yogurt, protein shakes, and smoothies.

- Drink nutrient-rich beverages instead of water and tea. Try hot chocolate, protein shakes, creamed soups, and nutritional supplements like Carnation Instant Breakfast, Ensure, Resurgex, and Boost.

ABOUT THE AUTHOR

Tinrin Chew, RD, CSO, is a registered dietitian who is board certified in oncology nutrition. She has twenty-seven years of medical-nutrition experience. During the past sixteen years, she has worked with cancer patients at the Alta Bates Summit Comprehensive Cancer Center in Berkeley, California. She also maintains her own private practice. She is a regular speaker for the Wellness Community and a lecturer for the Bay Area Tumor Institute. She has been coleading the "Navigating Through Chemotherapy and Nutrition" class at John Muir Medical Center and is involved in many local cancer support groups and education programs.

Chapter 8

Coping with Fatigue

It's common to hear people complain about feeling tired and worn out. The stress of living in a fast-paced, high-pressure, constantly changing world contributes to a sense of fatigue for many people. But for a person facing cancer and treatment, fatigue can take on a new meaning.

Before you began cancer treatment, your fatigue was probably just an occasional inconvenience, relieved with a good night's sleep. You were able to push past your feelings of exhaustion and carry on, despite feeling tired.

But when you're getting chemotherapy, fatigue can feel very different. During this time, you may not be able to push past your exhaustion to work or play as much as you did in the past. And catching up on your sleep may not relieve this feeling.

This chapter will explain why this level of fatigue can happen during chemotherapy. It will review medical treatments for fatigue that may work for you, and it will give you specific recommendations for how to manage it. Indeed, there are many things you can do to cope with fatigue.

WHY DOES FATIGUE HAPPEN?

There are many different reasons for the fatigue experienced by people receiving cancer treatment. To help you understand why you feel tired, here's a review of the possible causes.

Cancer

Cancer itself can cause fatigue. In fact, it can be one of the earliest symptoms of cancer. If you haven't received any treatment for cancer yet but are experiencing fatigue, this is probably why.

Cancer cells often reproduce more rapidly than normal cells, which requires a lot of energy, so a growing tumor can leave you feeling depleted and tired. Also, cancer sometimes causes fevers, which can make you feel tired and weak.

Depending on the type of cancer and its location, cancer can interfere with how well your body is functioning. If cancer is in the bone marrow, your body may not be able to make enough red blood cells to carry oxygen to each cell. If cancer is affecting your organs, your body may not be able to fully eliminate waste or absorb needed nutrients. Fatigue can also happen if cancer interferes with your ability to breathe because of a chronic cough, infection, fever, or fluid in your lungs. Anything that interrupts your body's normal functioning is likely to make you tired.

Treatments for Cancer

Many cancer treatments can also cause or contribute to fatigue. If you have surgery, chemotherapy, radiation therapy, or targeted therapies, you may notice some fatigue during treatment and while you recover from treatment.

SURGERY

If you had surgery to remove the cancer, it may take many weeks to regain your energy. The effects of general anesthesia take time to wear off. Your heart and lungs need time to recover. Your digestive system also needs time to recover from surgery, so you may not eat normally for a while and therefore may have less energy. Also, your muscles need time to recover, depending on how long you were in bed and inactive. Reduced mobility causes your muscles to lose strength and makes your fatigue worse.

Being in the hospital after surgery contributes to fatigue. It's often difficult to sleep in the hospital because it's an unfamiliar environment and often very noisy. Also, there are frequent interruptions of your sleep by hospital staff who awaken you to take your temperature and blood pressure, draw your blood, or give you medication.

CHEMOTHERAPY AND RADIATION THERAPY

Chemotherapy and radiation therapy kill cells that are reproducing rapidly. As cancer cells die, they create waste products. Your kidneys and liver have to work harder to eliminate these toxins, and that takes energy. Your body also has to work harder to replace the normal cells that have been affected by chemotherapy or radiation therapy, such as the lining of your digestive system and the blood-producing cells of your bone marrow.

TARGETED DRUG THERAPIES

Targeted therapies target cancer cells specifically. *Biological response modifiers* such as interferon or interleukin-2 help your own immune system combat the cancer by acting like naturally occurring substances in your body that fight diseases. Unfortunately, these treatments often cause flu-like symptoms that can result in fevers and fatigue. Other targeted therapies such as monoclonal antibodies can also make you feel tired. These are very specific antibodies that trigger your immune system to target and kill cancer cells.

Low Blood Counts

Your bone marrow contains cells that rapidly divide to produce new blood cells. You have three types of blood cells: red blood cells (RBCs) carry oxygen, white blood cells (WBCs) fight infection, and platelets make the blood clot to stop bleeding. Chemotherapy can affect your bone marrow and can cause a drop in the production of new blood cells (red cells, white cells, and platelets). Some chemotherapy drugs affect one type of blood cell more than the other types.

ANEMIA

Since red blood cells carry oxygen, a decrease in their number results in less oxygen going to all the cells in your body. Without enough oxygen, your cells are unable to perform normally. This causes fatigue and may also cause weakness or shortness of breath. Since red cells live a long time (about three to four months), you may not notice a decrease in red cells right away. But after several treatments you may experience fatigue, because they're not being replaced quickly enough by your bone marrow. That can make you feel more tired.

NEUTROPENIA

Neutrophils are the most common type of white blood cell. They're the first to fight infection. If cancer treatment inhibits your bone marrow from making enough new neutrophils, you can develop *neutropenia*, which means you don't have enough of these white cells in your blood to fight infection.

White cells, such as neutrophils, have a much shorter life span than red cells. They circulate in the bloodstream for only about twelve hours, so the number of these cells in your blood can decrease quickly—even after your first treatment. The time when your white-cell count is the lowest, the *nadir* (the low point), often occurs seven to ten days after each chemotherapy treatment. Many people report that they feel more fatigued during this time. Then when their white (neutrophil) count recovers, they have more energy.

Infection and Fever

At times during your cancer treatment, such as when your WBC count is low, you're more likely to get an infection. When that happens, your body will need to use more energy to fight the infection, and that can make you feel more tired.

Infections can also cause you to have a fever. An increase in your body temperature from fever makes your cells work harder and causes them to need more oxygen and nutrients. Your body works harder, which can make you more fatigued.

Pain

Anyone who experiences acute or chronic pain knows how exhausting it can be. It can limit your movement, appetite, sleep, and enjoyment of life. People in pain may be able to minimize the pain they feel during the day by using distraction. But this takes a lot of energy and can contribute to their fatigue.

Pain is often more noticeable at night and can interfere with sleep. Even if you spend eight hours in bed at night, you may toss and turn or wake up often. So your sleep may not be restful. If you don't sleep well, you won't have as much energy the next day.

Pain medicines are often sedating and can make you feel sleepy and tired during the day. Over time you may find this less of a problem as your body adjusts after a few days of taking the medication regularly.

Stress, Anxiety, and Sleep Disturbances

It's normal to worry and feel anxious when faced with a serious illness such as cancer. You may be concerned about many areas of your life, like your future, your family, your job, and your bills. These worries can be exhausting at times, particularly at night, and this can make it difficult for you to sleep.

In light of the many challenges someone with cancer faces, it's not unusual to feel overwhelmed, out of control, or depressed. These feelings usually come and go. You may feel down at times, but at other times you'll feel more positive. When you feel down, though, you're likely to feel more tired. Chapter 13 ("Mind and Body") addresses some of these concerns.

WHEN DOES FATIGUE HAPPEN?

You're likely to feel some fatigue throughout chemotherapy, though there may be periods when it can be more of a problem. The amount and intensity of fatigue may vary depending on the type and frequency of your treatments. Periods of fatigue usually occur at about the same time during each cycle of chemotherapy. Once you start treatment, you'll learn to anticipate your patterns of energy and fatigue. Then you'll be better able to plan activities, including your work schedule, personal commitments, and family events.

Your worst fatigue may be in the first day or two after each chemo treatment, when the chemicals are actively attacking cancer cells as well as some of your normal cells. You may not eat or drink normally. You may be taking medicines to prevent or relieve nausea that are sedating. And just coming to the clinic for your treatment can be stressful. So there are a number of reasons why you may feel wiped out. This is a good time to take it easy. Don't schedule anything more that would require a lot of energy.

If you receive a steroid hormone such as dexamethasone (Decadron) before or after your treatment, you may not feel tired at first. This is because the steroid can temporarily increase your sense of energy and appetite. It can also cause you to have trouble sleeping. Then, once it wears off, you may feel intense fatigue, as well as sadness and even depression, for a couple days as your body readjusts to normal hormone levels. Tell your doctor if either steroid-induced hyperactivity or depression is a problem for you. Sometimes the dose or schedule of the steroid can be adjusted to help with this.

You'll probably feel the most energy right before your next cycle of chemotherapy, because your body has had a chance to recover from your previous cycle.

HOW YOUR DOCTOR CAN HELP

If a low blood count, infection, fever, or pain contributes to your fatigue, your physician may be able to help. So talk to your physician or nurse about your level of fatigue and the impact it has on your life. Your experience of fatigue (like pain) is invisible to others and can't be measured as your blood pressure or your blood counts can. So they may have no way of knowing how tired you feel unless you tell them.

Anemia is one cause of fatigue that can be treated. If your physician suspects that you're anemic, she may order blood tests to check your iron levels. If your iron levels are low, you may need an iron supplement. Another treatment that may help you is an injection of a synthetic hormone, erythropoietin, which can stimulate your bone marrow to make more red blood cells (oxygen-carrying cells). You may not feel the effects of these treatments for several weeks, but eventually, as your iron levels or red cells increase, you'll have more energy. Severe anemia may require a transfusion of red blood cells to supplement the oxygen-carrying capacity of your blood until your bone marrow recovers. A transfusion can provide quick relief of anemia and fatigue. Your doctor will let you know if any of these treatments could be helpful to you.

Neutropenia (not enough white cells) can also be corrected by synthetic hormone injections to stimulate your bone marrow to make more neutrophils (infection-fighting cells). Short-acting and long-acting forms of this hormone are available. Your doctor will decide if you need it to help your bone marrow recover quickly, to lower the chance of getting an infection, and to be ready to get your next treatment on time. Once your neutrophil count returns to normal, you'll likely regain some energy.

Infection and fever are also conditions that can be treated. If you get an infection or fever during treatment, be sure to tell your physician or nurse. They may order tests (blood culture, urine culture, stool culture, chest X-ray) to determine the location and type of infection and start you on an antibiotic. When the infection resolves and your temperature returns to normal, your energy will improve.

Pain can also be treated. It's important to report any new pain, unrelieved pain, or change or increase in pain so that your doctor can evaluate the cause and provide relief. You may need a different pain medication or an adjustment or addition to your current pain medication to increase its effectiveness. This can greatly improve your sleep and reduce your fatigue.

THINGS YOU CAN DO

Although fatigue is inevitable at times during cancer treatment, there are many things you can do to minimize and cope with it. The following sections give you specific suggestions to increase or conserve your energy.

Exercise

Studies have shown that increased physical activity is a very effective way of managing fatigue during and following cancer treatment. It might not seem logical, but it's true. It really can help! That's because exercise increases muscle strength and improves heart and lung fitness. The more you exercise, the stronger your muscles, heart, and lungs get. If you're inactive, your muscles lose strength, making you feel more tired—which leads to more inactivity and more muscle weakness. Being physically active can break this cycle. Also, exercise has the added benefit of improving your appetite and sleep, and that can also give you more energy.

For those of you already exercising on a regular basis, keep it up. But be aware that you may run out of steam and may not be able to do as much or go as far as you did before treatment. Don't push yourself too hard. Listen to your body. You may need to slow down or rest more frequently.

If you haven't been exercising regularly and want to start, first talk to your physician or surgeon and ask whether there's any restriction on your activities and when it's safe to start an exercise program. After you get your physician's approval, start slowly with a low-impact exercise such as walking, swimming, cycling, or light weight training. Maybe all you'll be able to do at first is two minutes. That's okay. Keep that up on a regular basis (at least every other day) until you can do a little more. Then continue to slowly increase your exercise time.

Starting an exercise program can be difficult for anyone. You may feel so tired at times that exercising may seem too difficult, even if you know that it can be beneficial. Here are some suggestions to help you get started:

- Keep in mind that you need to balance your exercise with energy conservation. Rest when you're particularly tired, and exercise when you have periods of more energy. You'll learn when to expect these periods after your first cycle of chemo.

- Just taking a short walk for a few minutes can help you feel better, even the first day or two after your treatment.

- One way to ensure that you have time to exercise on a regular basis is to schedule it ahead of time on your calendar or daily planner. That will help prevent you from scheduling other activities at the same time or just forgetting about it altogether.

- It's easier to exercise if you make it enjoyable. So plan your exercise program based on what you enjoy. If you love being outdoors, choose an exercise you can do outdoors, like walking or swimming. If you like being with people, go to a gym or plan to get together with a friend for a walk or bike ride in the neighborhood.

- If the thought of leaving home to exercise doesn't appeal to you, there are DVDs or CDs you can follow right in your living room.

- Whatever type of exercise you choose, reward yourself for sticking with it. You might keep an exercise calendar and make a notation each time you exercise as an ongoing record of your accomplishments. Then, when you achieve your goal for the week, find a way to reward yourself.

Conserve Your Energy and Manage Your Activities

Most people already have such busy lives these days that it's a challenge just to manage all of their activities and commitments.

When you're getting cancer treatment, it may be an even bigger challenge managing your time because of the extra time required for medical appointments, paperwork, and phone calls. So it's important to conserve your energy and manage your time well. Here are some tips.

Prioritize. Evaluate and prioritize your activities. Low-priority activities can be reassigned to another day or to someone else. Eliminate the activities that aren't truly important. Don't try to do it all. You just won't have the energy. Make time to be with friends or family who make you feel good. Many people say that it sometimes helps to focus on something else besides cancer or treatments. If possible, keep doing the things you enjoy and that make you feel "normal."

Schedule. Plan and schedule your activities during your high-energy periods. Pace yourself, and don't try to do too much at once. Listen to your body. When you start to feel tired, rest. Don't push yourself until you have no energy left. If needed, change or cancel your plans. It helps to alternate an activity or a project with a rest period. After taking a break, you'll be able to resume the activity with more energy and enthusiasm.

Be efficient. Don't waste your time or energy. Make a list before you go to the store so that you don't forget something and have to go back. At the store, use a cart with wheels rather than a handheld basket to carry items. Some grocery stores have banking services and postal services on site; some stores will deliver your purchases to your home. If you can shop by catalog or online, you'll save yourself the effort needed to drive, park, walk through crowded malls, and carry heavy bags.

Ask for help, and be specific. Other people may not be aware of the kind of fatigue you're experiencing. This is especially true if the fatigue is intermittent: some days you feel fine, and other days you need more help or more rest. So it's important to communicate how you feel and what others can do to help you. Involve your family, friends, and coworkers. It's okay to ask for help and delegate tasks.

People are often anxious to help but just don't know how. Be clear with them about exactly what help you need. When you're specific, you're more likely to get the help you want.

Use community resources. In many communities, there are resources (both public and private) that can help you manage some of the routine errands that take energy. For example, there are agencies that deliver home-cooked meals at a cost based on your income. There are volunteers who drive people to and from the clinic or hospital for appointments or chemo treatments. Your social worker or nurse can tell you about other community resources that may be of help to you.

Improve Your Sleep

Sleep is important for everyone, but it's especially important while you're getting cancer treatments. Sleep allows your body and mind to recover and heal from the stress. What can seem overwhelming when you're exhausted may seem less so if you had slept well the night before.

There are several ways you can help yourself fall asleep more easily and avoid waking up before morning so that you get a good night's sleep.

Sleep schedule. Maintaining a regular sleep schedule is important for a good night of sleep. This means going to bed and getting up at approximately the same time every day. Also taking naps earlier in the day and limiting them to thirty to forty minutes will make it easier for you to fall asleep at night.

Exercise. Regular exercise improves your sleep. But it's best to exercise at least three hours before bedtime so that your body and mind have a chance to settle down before sleep.

Relaxation. Going to bed feeling relaxed helps you to fall asleep. So allow yourself one to two hours to relax each night before bedtime. Taking a warm bath or shower, reading a good book, listening to soft music, and receiving a massage are some good ways to feel relaxed and sleepy. Reading or doing craft work before sleep works as well. Avoid watching overstimulating TV or movies just before sleep. They may keep you awake, still feeling excited or anxious, long after the show is over. Try different activities and find what works for you.

Bedtime snacks. Avoid stimulants such as coffee, tea, and chocolate after noon. Alcohol, especially at bedtime, can also keep you awake. Eat dinner at least three hours before going to bed so that your body has time to digest your food. But don't go to bed hungry; eat a light snack. A good choice is crackers with cheese or warm milk, because they contain chemicals (tryptophan and serotonin) that help your brain to relax.

Environment. There are also things you can do to make your bedroom more conducive to sleep. Make sure you have a comfortable bed in a secure, quiet room. Adjust the temperature so that it's cool rather than warm, and adjust the window coverings so that sunlight or streetlights are blocked. Get rid of any clutter, work-related papers, unused hospital supplies, and other things that may distract you from relaxation and sleep.

Eat Well

Your body needs adequate nutrition to help your cells recover and to give you energy. But there may be things that make that difficult.

Are you nauseated or vomiting? Have you lost your appetite? Do you feel full even though you've eaten very little? Are you having trouble chewing or swallowing? Or are you too tired to cook a nutritious meal? If you have any of these problems, you may not be eating enough food to provide the fuel your body needs to heal itself and give you energy. So it's important for you to identify and eliminate as many of these obstacles as possible. Talk to your physician, nurse, or nutritionist for help.

Nausea and vomiting. If you have nausea or vomiting, be sure you're taking the antinausea medications the way they were prescribed. If the medications aren't working for you, tell your physician or nurse so that your medication can be changed or adjusted. Relieving nausea, especially before you eat, is essential. Chapter 5 ("Preventing Nausea") provides many more ideas about how to prevent and relieve the nausea associated with cancer treatments.

Lack of appetite. If you have no appetite or feel full quickly after eating a small amount of food, try preparing smaller portions of food at each meal. In addition to these smaller meals, eat three or four nutritious snacks between your meals and at bedtime. You can also add more nutrition to your diet with liquid supplements, which are high in calories, protein, vitamins, and other nutrients. These supplements are also good if you have trouble chewing or swallowing food. Try different brands and flavors to find the ones you like best.

Fatigue. If there are days when you're too tired to cook a healthy meal, prepare and freeze food on the days when you have more energy. Divide it into meal-sized portions so that you can easily defrost and eat it on days when you're too tired to make dinner. You can also enlist the help of family, friends, or neighbors. Ask one friend to organize the people who want to help so that they take turns bringing you dinner on the days when you need them. Be sure to let them know your dietary restrictions and what you can eat and enjoy during this time. Your taste and preferences may be different than before.

Get Support

Sometimes just talking to others who are also experiencing fatigue can be beneficial. It can be helpful to know that you aren't the only person struggling with low energy. Also, many people are happy to share with you what they've found helpful in dealing with fatigue, stress, or sleep difficulties.

You may meet people who are getting chemo at the same time as you. They're often happy to share their experiences. A cancer support group is also a good way to meet other people who are getting, or who've completed, cancer treatment. The support-group members provide support to each other and share ideas and suggestions they've found to be helpful. If there are no support groups near you, a local American Cancer Society (ACS) office may be able to connect you to a cancer survivor who can be a resource and support.

IN CONCLUSION

When we feel well, it may seem that our energy is limitless. We can push ourselves and go without sleep when necessary to accomplish what we need or want to do. But when going through cancer-fighting treatments, you may experience energy as a finite quantity. There are days when you have more or less of it. At times you'll need to slow down and make changes in your activities. Be patient, rest, and eat well. Give yourself time to recover, and your energy will return.

Chapter 9

Coping with Hair Loss and Skin Changes

Most of the temporary changes caused by the side effects of chemotherapy happen inside your body. They aren't obvious to others. You can't see a low white-blood-cell count or changes in appetite or digestion. But changes in your hair and skin happen on the outside of your body, so they're visible to others. Therefore, many people find that cancer treatment's effect on their appearance is very stressful. The way you wear your hair is one of the ways you express your identity and individual style. So dealing with hair loss or thinning can be a difficult or even traumatic adjustment, although these changes are temporary. Changes in your skin or nails can affect your comfort, appearance, mobility, and activity level.

Your doctor or nurse will tell you about the changes in hair and skin that you can anticipate from your particular treatment. As with the other potential side effects of treatment, if you know what to expect, you'll be better prepared to cope with any problems. This chapter will explain how chemotherapy can affect your hair, skin, and nails and what you can do to cope with the changes during this time.

HAIR

Chemotherapy works by damaging cells that are rapidly dividing. As a result, cancer cells, which divide frequently, are extremely vulnerable to the effects of chemotherapy. But the normal cells in your body, some of which also divide frequently, can be temporarily damaged. Since chemotherapy travels via your bloodstream to every cell in your body, your hair can be affected.

Hair grows from follicles embedded deep inside your skin or scalp. Since at any one time, about 90 percent of your hair follicles are in the active growth phase, they're especially susceptible to the effects of chemotherapy. Hair loss occurs when chemotherapy damages dividing follicle cells, producing weak, brittle hair that may break off at the scalp or fall out at the root itself. And it's not only the hair on your head that may be affected by chemotherapy. Some people notice that their eyebrows are thinner and they have fewer eyelashes. Also, some people lose hair on their arms, legs, and pubic area. But in general, since the hair on the rest of your body doesn't grow as rapidly as the hair on your head, you may not notice significant hair loss in these other areas due to chemotherapy.

Whether or not you lose your hair depends on the type and dosage of the chemotherapy drugs you receive. Some drugs may not affect your hair at all. Some may cause partial hair loss (hair thinning). And some chemotherapy drugs will cause complete hair loss. The newer, "targeted" drugs usually don't cause any hair loss. That's because they don't affect all rapidly dividing cells in your body. Your doctor or nurse will tell you what to expect from the specific drugs and dosages you're getting.

Hair Loss

Although damage to hair follicles from chemotherapy is immediate, you won't see the result of that damage until at least two weeks later. Your scalp may feel very sensitive, itchy, or tingly at first. Then you may notice unusually large amounts of hair coming out on your brush or pillow, or find more hair in the shower drain.

As more hair shafts break and less hair grows in because of the damage to the hair follicles, the remaining hair on your head will appear thinner. In some cases hair loss will show up in patches.

Just like the cells of your digestive system or bone marrow, damaged hair follicles recover quickly from the effects of chemotherapy. They start producing hair again, but because hair grows slowly, you probably won't notice hair growth before your next chemotherapy treatment, when the cycle is repeated. People who receive chemotherapy treatments monthly or more often usually won't see hair growth begin to return until about a month or two after all chemotherapy treatments are completed.

Coping with Hair Loss

Even when people expect to lose their hair from chemotherapy, it's still upsetting when it actually happens. Since there's a delay of a couple weeks from the beginning of treatments to when the hair starts to fall out, you most likely won't be in the clinic when it happens. So you won't have the support of nurses or other medical staff who are familiar with what's happening to you.

It's distressing to see your hair clogging the drain or filling the brush. If your hair is long, it may be helpful to have it cut into a shorter style even before starting the treatment that will cause hair loss. Some people even shave their heads before it starts to fall out.

It may help to talk to someone else who has experienced hair loss. You can talk to other people in the clinic or in a cancer support group. Also, don't hesitate to check back in with the nurse at your oncologist's office for support or suggestions. Keep in mind that hair loss from chemotherapy is temporary. Your hair will regrow after your treatments are over.

ABOUT WIGS

If you plan to get a wig, it may be helpful to take some photographs of your hairline and your hairstyle from the front, side, and back. Snip little samples of your hair from the front and back as well. Then you can match the wig's texture, color, and style to your own hair.

Purchase your wig from a store that can provide experienced sales staff, privacy, and individual attention. If you're unsure about where to go, ask your nurse or the American Cancer Society for a referral. Or a member of your support group may recommend a particular store or salesperson who's been especially helpful.

In order to buy a wig that's as natural-looking and comfortable as possible, there are a number of things to consider when shopping.

Type of wig. Synthetic and human-hair wigs each have advantages. Many women prefer synthetic wigs, because they're easier to maintain and much less expensive. Synthetic "hair" ranges from stiff to almost silky. Some women prefer human-hair wigs because of their natural feel and versatility. You can restyle a human-hair wig as often as real hair and touch it up using a curling iron or blow-dryer that would melt a synthetic wig.

Wig construction. The way a wig is constructed affects its comfort and how natural it looks. If the wig has a vented cap, it will be more comfortable. More expensive custom-made wigs have hair that is implanted into a skin-like base. They're more comfortable and look more natural.

Fit. It's very important that the wig fit you well. If you're constantly aware of it or if you're afraid to move in a natural way because it's uncomfortable, then you won't feel good wearing it. Buying a wig while you still have some hair can be a problem, because it may not fit as well after all your hair is gone. Be sure to have the wig refitted if necessary to assure comfort and the most natural look. There are usually hooks or Velcro in the back that can be adjusted for a better fit.

Comfort. Your body generates heat, and when you perspire, the air evaporates the moisture you've generated to cool you down. You might not normally notice the perspiration from your head, but it can be a problem when you wear a wig. If the air isn't able to reach your scalp, you may notice the perspiration making your scalp itch or feel hot. This can make your wig uncomfortable. To overcome the problem, try wrapping a thin cotton scarf around your head under the wig. Or, you can get a piece of stretch stockinette material that can be tied at one end to make a cap. This can then be worn under the wig, helping to absorb perspiration as well as providing a cushion between your wig and your scalp.

Cost. The prices of wigs vary greatly. The cost may be covered by your insurance if the doctor writes a prescription for a "cranial prosthesis." (*Prosthesis* is the medical term for the replacement of a missing part by an artificial substitute.) The prescription must also indicate the medical necessity for the wig, for example, "Alopecia (hair loss) due to chemotherapy." Most physicians are aware of the wording required for your insurance company to reimburse you for the cost of your wig. If your insurance can offset some of the cost of the wig, you may be able to afford a more expensive one that's more comfortable and more natural looking.

ALTERNATIVES TO A WIG

In addition to wigs, there are hats and head wraps with hair attached. The hair may show from under the hat or head wrap as bangs, a fall, or a ponytail. These coverings can give the illusion of a full head of hair.

Many women use scarves and head wraps as alternatives to wearing a wig. It's a way to add color, texture, and accents to your wardrobe. A basic cotton square folded into two uneven triangles and tied at the back of your neck can be both colorful and comfortable. You can add a contrasting color by twisting another scarf or cord and tying that around the first scarf. You can also experiment with side knots or adding a hat or beret over the scarf.

In your own home or for sleep, you might try a soft terry-cloth or cotton turban. It's an easy and comfortable alternative to a wig or head wrap.

Baseball caps are often used by both men and women. They're colorful and can be worn either with or without a head wrap.

If you choose not to use any head covering, you need to be aware of the weather and the sun. Hair serves as an insulation, to protect your body from losing heat. In cold weather you can become chilled easily, so you'll need a hat or scarf when outdoors. Your hair also protects your scalp from the ultraviolet rays of the sun, so you'll need a hat or sunscreen (at least SPF 15) while you're in direct sunlight to avoid sunburn. Remember, the sun can cause a burn even in cool weather or when the sky is overcast.

HOW TO COPE WITH THINNING HAIR

Many cancer treatments cause your hair to become dry and brittle, and can make it appear to be thinner than before. When your hair is more fragile, you should be especially gentle in your hair care. Here are some suggestions:

- Wash and dry your hair gently; it's even more fragile when wet.

- Check with your barber or hairdresser for special products designed for "overtreated" or "damaged" hair.

- Avoid harsh chemicals like peroxide or permanent solutions.

- Don't use a hot blow-dryer or hot curlers. They'll make your hair even dryer and more likely to break.

- Many people find that shorter hair camouflages hair thinning. Longer hair is heavier, and the weight pulls it flatter on your head. Hair that's shorter tends to spring upward, contributing to a fuller look.

- If your hair is long, you may want to cut it a little at a time. The change won't be so drastic, and you'll have a chance to adjust gradually to a different look.

- Don't forget the importance of eating a well-balanced diet to keep your hair healthy. Poor nutrition due to nausea or a diminished appetite may contribute to dull and lifeless hair.

Regrowth of Hair

When your hair returns, at first it will feel like peach fuzz. Later you may notice other differences in texture. If your hair was curly before, your new hair may grow in straighter. Previously straight hair may grow in curly. Your hair may be finer or coarser than it was before, and your hair may grow in darker or lighter than your natural color. But if your hair grows back differently at first, over time it may return to its original color and texture.

SKIN AND NAILS

Like your hair, your skin and nails may be affected by chemotherapy. Your doctor will tell you what changes you can expect during your treatment.

Dryness

Dry skin can be caused by a number of different factors: the effects of chemotherapy, antinausea medication, dehydration, or poor nutrition. It's not only uncomfortable and itchy, it's also more likely to be damaged by normal activities. Here are some suggestions to prevent and treat dry, itchy skin:

- Use a moisturizing soap to prevent the drying effects of regular soap.

- Take warm, rather than hot, baths or showers. Hot water can actually dry your skin.

- Pat your skin dry with a soft towel. Don't rub.

- After washing, lubricate your skin well with a water-based moisturizer.

- Avoid scented and other alcohol-based products, because they'll dry your skin.

- Avoid letting wool or other scratchy fabrics come in contact with your skin. Cotton is more comfortable.

- Soft, loose clothing is less irritating than tight-fitting clothing, which may bind or cause more irritation to skin that's already dry.

- Wear gloves in cold weather to protect your hands.

- Use a skin lubricant such as Bag Balm or Udderly Smooth to heal severely dry, cracked skin. These products are available without a prescription.

Sunburn

Some chemotherapy drugs will make your skin more sensitive to the sun. This means that sun exposure that would ordinarily not affect you could cause a burn. If the chemotherapy drugs you receive cause increased sun sensitivity, take precautions. Use sunscreen with a protection level of at least SPF 15. Be generous with sunscreen on areas likely to be exposed to the sun, such as your face, neck, shoulders, and ankles. Use lip gloss or lip balm with sunscreen to protect your lips. Wear a hat with a brim wide enough to protect your face and neck, as well as long sleeves and long pants to protect your arms and legs. Remember that even on hazy days, the sun's rays can penetrate to cause a burn.

Tanning

The color of your skin is the result of the amount of *melanin* it contains. Dark-skinned people have more melanin than light-skinned people. Your pituitary gland produces a melanin-stimulating hormone (MSH) that determines your complexion. When you're exposed to the sun, your pituitary is stimulated to produce more melanin, thus bringing about the normal tanning process.

Some chemotherapy drugs stimulate your body to make more melanin than usual, and as a result your skin may temporarily become darker. Since these drugs travel through the bloodstream to every part of your body, they can cause a generalized tanning effect evenly distributed over your body, like a regular suntan.

Sometimes the tanning effect is most visible as a darkening in your nail beds (the skin under your nails), on the skin over your joints, or in the mucous membranes of your mouth. If you're getting chemotherapy into the veins of your hands or arms, you may develop a darkening in the skin over those veins. It may seem that the patterns of the veins in your hands or arms are outlined in a color several shades darker than your normal skin tone. If you're getting chemotherapy into larger veins near your heart through a VAD, you won't see this darkening pattern over the veins. People with darker skin may be more likely to develop the darkening effect than people with lighter skin.

Your doctor or nurse will tell you if your chemotherapy is likely to cause tanning or sun sensitivity. Just remember that the tanning or darkening caused by some chemotherapy drugs is temporary. You may notice it beginning two to three weeks after the start of treatment, and it will start to fade away after all your treatments are completed.

Flushing

Your skin may become temporarily flushed for a few days after receiving some chemotherapy drugs. This redness is caused by dilation of blood vessels. Most of the time, the flushing will occur in a localized area, usually on your face or neck. This flushing isn't painful, although the redness can be fairly bright. Unlike the tanning effect, which can last for a long time, flushing will usually disappear a few days after your treatment. Your doctor or nurse will tell you if you're getting a chemotherapy drug that's likely to cause flushing.

Acne-Like Rash

Some of the "targeted" chemotherapy drugs work by blocking signals to specific receptors on the surface of cancer cells. This type of treatment is meant to stop the cancer cells from growing. These receptors are called *epidermal growth factor receptors* (*EGFRs*), and the drugs are called *anti-epidermal growth factor receptor* (*anti-EGFR*) drugs. Cetuximab (Erbitux), gefitinib (Iressa), and erlotinib (Tarceva) are examples of this kind of targeted therapy.

Because these receptors are also found on normal skin cells, people getting this type of treatment can develop a rash on the face, neck, or chest that may look like acne. This can occur a week or two after starting treatment. The rash can make your skin look red and feel dry and itchy or painful. Let your doctor know if you're developing this rash. Don't try to treat it yourself with acne medications, because they'll make your skin even dryer, which can make the rash worse.

Your doctor may prescribe a topical antibiotic and a soothing moisturizer to promote healing. Some people may need to take an oral antibiotic if the rash is severe.

Here are some suggestions to help you if you have this rash:

- Use a mild soap to avoid irritating your skin.

- Use hypoallergenic, unscented moisturizer daily to prevent or relieve dryness.

- Use hypoallergenic makeup, if desired, to cover up the rash.

- Avoid sun exposure or tanning salons, which can worsen the redness.

- Don't use commercial acne medications. They can worsen dry and peeling skin.

Hand-Foot Syndrome

Some chemotherapy drugs such as capecitabine (Xeloda) and liposomal doxorubicin (Doxil) can cause the skin on the palms of your hands and soles of your feet to become red, tender, or swollen. This is called *hand-foot syndrome*. Usually this is a mild reaction that improves over a week or two. If the symptoms persist or become severe, you may need to take a break from the chemotherapy drug, resume the drug at a different dose or schedule, or change to a different drug.

Early signs of hand-foot syndrome include tingling, burning, itching, redness, and dryness. If these symptoms progress, you can develop peeling skin, swelling, and blisters. Tell your physician or nurse if you start to get any of these symptoms. They may recommend or prescribe a salve to promote healing and comfort. Treatments for hand-foot syndrome include cooling measures such as cold baths and ice packs, commercial creams (Bag Balm or Udderly Smooth), and a prescription cream (Biafine) that contains a combination of medications to promote comfort and healing.

If you're getting a chemotherapy drug that can cause hand-foot syndrome, here are some tips to help you prevent this reaction:

- Use a mild soap.

- Avoid lotions and creams that contain perfume, alcohol, or glycerin. Also, avoid numbing medicines, steroids such as hydrocortisone, and antihistamines such as diphenhydramine (Benadryl) unless instructed by your doctor.

- Stay out of direct sunlight.

- Protect your hands and feet from hot water. Don't use whirlpools, spas, or heated pools, and avoid using hot water for showers, washing dishes, or doing laundry.

- Wear comfortable, well-ventilated, nonbinding shoes or slippers. Wear socks to prevent irritation.

- Try not to put pressure on the palms of your hands (such as from carrying heavy objects, chopping hard foods, and gardening). Avoid pressure on the soles of your feet from walking or standing for long periods.

Radiation Recall

If you're receiving chemotherapy at the same time as or shortly after getting radiation therapy, you may develop red or dry peeling skin in the area that was radiated. This effect is called *radiation recall*. It may be caused by the chemotherapy's interfering with the repair of radiation-damaged skin cells.

If this happens, you should consult with your doctor or nurse in the radiation department. They may prescribe an ointment to promote healing. It's always wise to treat the affected skin gently by using mild soap and avoiding irritating clothing and exposure to the sun. Avoid extremes in heat (heating pad, hot-water bottle, or hot showers) or cold (ice packs or exposure to cold wind). If the symptoms are severe, you may have to take a break from chemotherapy until your skin improves.

Allergic Skin Reactions

At any time—not just during cancer treatments—you can have an allergic skin reaction to a particular medicine, food, or irritant. An allergic skin reaction may appear as raised, red, or itchy bumps on your skin. If this happens, you should check with your doctor or nurse as soon as possible. The itchiness of an allergic skin reaction can be quite irritating, and if untreated it may cause infection or other skin problems.

Sometimes it's obvious what caused the allergic reaction, and you can prevent it from happening again. If you get a skin reaction immediately after starting a new medication or eating a certain food, you can guess that it may be the source of the problem. Sometimes, however, it's difficult to determine what exactly is causing the problem. You can develop an allergic reaction to a medication or food that you may have tolerated well in the past. You can develop an allergic reaction after working in the yard or wearing clothes washed with your usual detergent. Sometimes you'll never be able to determine with certainty what has caused the problem.

Be sure to report any allergic skin reaction to your doctor or nurse. You may need an antihistamine or steroid to stop the allergic reaction and bring relief.

Nail Changes

Your nails grow from under the skin at the base of your cuticle. Chemotherapy's effect on these cells can cause your nails to become brittle and grow at a slower rate than usual or to become very soft, making them more likely to tear. After several weeks, when the part of your nail that was under your cuticle when you got your chemotherapy grows out to where it's visible, you may see a white or dark band or ridge in the nail. As your nail continues to grow and the band or ridge moves closer to the tip of your finger, you may find that the nail breaks more easily, peels, or catches on your clothing.

To prevent your nails from tearing, you should clip them close to your fingertips. Protect your nails and don't put added stress on them that may cause them to break. For example, don't use your nails to open soda cans. Some people find that tape or Band-Aids effectively prevent snagging while that fragile band or ridge grows out. Your nails are the best protection against pain or infection in the nail beds, so try to let the ridges grow out naturally without peeling them off early and exposing the nail bed to damage.

Don't use artificial nails during chemotherapy. If moisture collects under the artificial nail, you can develop a fungal infection that's hard to treat. You should also not use alcohol-based polish or polish remover, because these will make your nails drier and more likely to break and peel. Only use polish remover that's lanolin-based.

IN CONCLUSION

Appearance and body image are important to most people. So it's good to have help to cope with the temporary changes in your appearance caused by cancer treatments. A number of resources offer help so that you can look better and feel better about yourself.

The American Cancer Society has put together a program called "Look Good, Feel Better." Specially trained cosmetologists teach classes to help people with changes in their appearance from chemotherapy. These classes offer tips for applying makeup, wearing scarves creatively, and camouflaging skin changes. Ask your nurse or call 1-800-395-LOOK to see if there's a class available near you. The website www.lookgoodfeelbetter.org also offers helpful tips for dealing with hair loss and skin problems due to chemotherapy.

Chapter 10

Coping with Nervous-System Changes

You move through and experience the world by means of your nervous system. Your ability to think, remember, see, hear, taste, smell, touch, and move depends on the nerve fibers that send electrical signals throughout your body. This chapter will tell you about two possible side effects of chemotherapy that can affect your nervous system: peripheral neuropathy and "chemo brain." Here's some information about how your nervous system works.

Your brain and spinal cord form the *central nervous system*. All the other nerves that branch out from your spinal cord are part of the *peripheral nervous system*.

The basic component of your nervous system is the nerve cell called a *neuron*. Neurons are electrically excitable cells that process and transmit signals to your whole body: eyes and ears, muscles, organs, and skin. A neuron is made up of a star-shaped *cell body*, which receives information, and a long, thin, cable-like tail called an *axon*, which transmits information away from the cell body. These neurons can vary greatly in size. The neurons in your brain and spinal cord can be very tiny. Some axons can be very long; the longest ones can be three feet long and extend from the base of your spine to the tips of your toes.

Motor neurons carry signals from your brain to your muscles, enabling you to move your body. *Sensory neurons* carry signals from your sensory receptors (for sight, hearing, taste, and so on) back to your brain.

PERIPHERAL NEUROPATHY

We've all experienced numbness or tingling in an arm or a leg when it has "fallen asleep." It may have felt "dead," or maybe it felt like "pins and needles." The feeling probably went away quickly when you changed your position and your circulation returned to normal. But the feeling of numbness and tingling associated with some chemotherapy medicines is not caused by circulation or position. It's caused by the effect these medicines can have on nerve cells. The medical term for this condition is *peripheral neuropathy*. Your doctor will let you know if your treatment can cause this problem.

Peripheral neuropathy refers to the distortion or interruption in the normal flow of signals through the neurons that can affect movement or sensation. Other conditions or medical problems, such as injury, diabetes, circulation problems, kidney disease, and nutritional deficits can also cause neuropathy. Peripheral neuropathy caused by chemotherapy is often temporary and resolves over a period of weeks to months after treatment. Sometimes there are residual effects that can last longer.

It's not completely understood how chemotherapy can injure peripheral nerves. Some chemo drugs appear to damage the tail end (axon) of nerve cells. The most vulnerable axons are often the longest ones, which are those that extend to the toes and fingers. Later, if symptoms progress, they may be felt in the feet, ankles, or hands. When the chemotherapy drug is stopped, nerve cells may recover and grow new axons over time.

There are two types of peripheral neuropathy. The more common type is called *sensory*, because it affects the nerves needed for touch, temperature, and pain. The symptoms of this type are numbness, tingling (pins and needles), pain, and loss of feeling. This usually occurs in the hands and feet, and sometimes in the jaw. The less common type of peripheral neuropathy is called *motor*, because it's caused by a disruption of signals to the muscles. This can cause weakness, clumsiness, balance problems, foot drop (difficulty lifting your foot), or wrist drop (difficulty lifting your hand).

Several types of chemotherapy drugs can cause peripheral neuropathy. Two of the most common classes of drugs that can cause these problems are the *taxanes*, such as paclitaxel (Taxol) and docetaxel (Taxotere), and *platinum drugs*, such as cisplatin (Platinol) and oxaliplatin (Eloxatin). The taxanes and platinum drugs are primarily associated with the sensory type of neuropathy, usually experienced as numbness, tingling, or burning pain that can start in the fingers and toes but may progress to the hands and feet.

Some people may experience mild numbness or tingling for a day or two after each treatment, but they usually find that these symptoms go away in a few days. For some people these symptoms may persist longer and become more noticeable. It's important to let your doctor know:

- What symptoms you're having (numbness, pain, difficulty with movement, balance problems, and so on)

- What part of your body is affected

- How long these symptoms last; when are the symptoms better? When are they are worse?

- If they interfere with your activities, comfort, or sleep

If you start to experience neuropathy, your physician may slow down your chemo infusion or change the dose or frequency of your treatments. If you're experiencing a lot of neuropathy and it's getting worse, your doctor may switch to a different chemotherapy that doesn't cause this problem.

Cold Sensitivity

If you receive the platinum drug oxaliplatin (Eloxatin), you're also likely to notice a different kind of sensory neuropathy. It occurs when you come in contact with cold temperatures. This can happen if your body gets cold, if you touch something cold, or if you eat or drink something cold. These symptoms usually last for only a few days after each treatment. Here are some suggestions to help you manage while you're experiencing temporary cold sensitivity:

- Cover yourself with a blanket during your treatment.

- Wear warm clothing at all times in cold weather.

- Don't run the air-conditioning at high levels in the house or car.

- Take a warm shower.

- In cold weather, cover your mouth and nose with a scarf or ski cap to warm the air that you breathe. Don't breathe deeply when out in cold air.

- Wear gloves (or oven mitts) when you take things from the freezer or refrigerator.

- Wear gloves to touch cold objects, especially metal, such as your car door or mailbox.

- Only drink fluids and eat foods that are at room temperature or warmer (even ice cream).

- Avoid ice chips and ice cubes.

- If your body gets cold, warm it up quickly. If your hands get cold, wash them in warm water.

Things that Can Help Peripheral Neuropathy

There are various remedies to soothe symptoms of peripheral neuropathy and encourage regeneration of the injured nerves. These remedies include nutritional supplements, medications, acupuncture, physical therapy, and gentle massage. You may need to try different things to find what works for you. Sometimes a combination of methods is needed to help relieve the numbness and tingling or pain.

Nutritional supplements. Some nutritional supplements can help you to prevent or alleviate symptoms of neuropathy. One that's commonly used during treatment with the taxanes paclitaxel (Taxol) and docetaxel (Taxotere) is glutamine. *Glutamine* is an amino acid (protein building block) that's normally produced by your body. During periods of high stress, however, the body can't produce enough to meet its needs. Glutamine seems to protect the peripheral nerves from injury during chemo. It's often taken three or four times a day for several days after each taxane treatment to prevent or reduce the severity of symptoms.

Another nutritional supplement called *alpha-lipoic acid* has been helpful in preventing and relieving peripheral neuropathy. Alpha-lipoic acid is an antioxidant produced naturally by the body. It's also found in some foods, such as spinach, broccoli, peas, brussels sprouts, and rice bran. It's been shown to relieve symptoms of peripheral neuropathy in people with diabetes.

For more information about nutritional supplements during chemotherapy, talk to a nutritionist who specializes in oncology. Before taking any nutritional supplement during chemo, always check with your physician.

Medications. There are medications that can help if your symptoms are painful. Some of these are primarily used for treating other medical conditions, but they've been found to work for painful neuropathy symptoms.

Anticonvulsants and antidepressants have been helpful in providing relief. Gabapentin (Neurontin) helps calm the peripheral nerves. Some antidepressants, such as amitriptyline (Elavil) and venlafaxine (Effexor), decrease the chemicals in the brain that transmit pain signals. Both anticonvulsants and antidepressants are used at much lower doses to treat peripheral neuropathy than to treat depression or convulsions. You may start at a low dose and then increase over time if needed.

Mild pain relievers like acetaminophen (Tylenol) and anti-inflammatory pain relievers like ibuprofen (Motrin, Advil) may be useful for painful neuropathy symptoms. You may need stronger medication, such as hydrocodone or oxycodone. These pain medications may be prescribed alone or in combination with an anticonvulsant or an antidepressant to get the most benefit.

Acupuncture. This traditional practice has been used successfully to relieve pain from peripheral neuropathy. It's an ancient Chinese technique that uses very thin needles inserted into the body at certain energy points. Stimulating these points activates and balances the vital energy or life force, called *chi* (pronounced "chee"), which travels in the body through a system of energy channels called *meridians*.

According to Western medicine, acupuncture likely works by stimulating the central nervous system (brain and spinal cord) to release neurotransmitters and hormones. These chemicals control sensation, such as pain; boost the immune system; and regulate various body functions, such as blood pressure.

Physical therapy. This therapy may reduce weakness and clumsiness caused by peripheral neuropathy. Through range-of-motion and stretching exercises, physical therapy may strengthen weak muscles, increase circulation, and improve balance and coordination. Physical therapists can teach you exercises that you can do at home. Your doctor can make a referral to a physical therapy clinic for treatment.

Gentle massage. Sometimes called "bodywork," massage can increase circulation and promote relaxation. It's sometimes useful in providing relief from the symptoms of neuropathy as well. Check with your physician before having a massage. If you ever find massage painful, don't continue.

Safety Measures

If you have numbness or tingling in your hands or feet, it's important for you to maintain healthy skin. You may have decreased sensation and be unable to feel the discomfort that would normally alert you to a problem like a cut or a burn. Here are some recommendations to help you take extra-good care of your skin:

- Inspect your hands and feet daily for sores, cuts, burns, or blisters.

- Avoid ill-fitting or tight shoes and socks.

- Moisturize your hands and feet daily and massage them gently.

- Be sure to dry in between toes after bathing, to avoid fungal infections.

- Keep toenails carefully trimmed to avoid infection or injury. If this is difficult for you or your toes are numb, your doctor can refer you to a podiatrist for this care.

- Wear warm socks and gloves during cold weather. Hands and feet can become more painful with cold temperatures.

- Use rubber gloves when washing dishes to avoid burns and cuts and to help you hold on to slippery plates if you have numbness in your fingers.

- Lower the temperature in your home water heater to less than 120 degrees to avoid burns. You may not be able to feel if the water is too hot.

If your neuropathy is causing numbness, weakness, or clumsiness, you may be at risk for falls or other accidents around the house. To prevent falls, you should use commonsense safety measures such as the following:

- Make sure the lights are on when entering a room.

- Use a lighted key ring to open locked doors. You may not be able to "feel" the keyhole when your fingers are numb.

- Remove throw rugs. They can cause slips and falls.

- Clear walkways of clutter, toys, and other objects to avoid tripping.

- Wear sturdy shoes. Avoid slippers or athletic shoes with very thick soles.

- Use skid-free shower and bath mats, and install hand-rails in the bath or shower.

PERIPHERAL NEUROPATHY AND CONSTIPATION

Your large intestine (colon) is responsible for absorbing fluid. It does that by moving the fluid-food mixture from your small intestine (where digestion takes place) through the length of the colon until you pass a soft, solid stool. If the large intestine moves the mixture through too fast, you'll have liquid or loose stools. If it moves it through too slowly, you'll have hard stools that are difficult to pass. The longer the food-fluid mixture sits in the colon, the more water is extracted and the harder the stool becomes.

Many things, such as medications, toxins, diet, activity, and stress, can affect the normal movement through the intestines (*peristalsis*).

There are peripheral nerves that control the normal waves of movement through your large intestine. A class of chemotherapy drugs called *vinca alkaloids*, including vincristine (Oncovin) and vinblastine (Velban), can affect these peripheral nerves. The result is a slowing of the gastrointestinal system, which can lead to constipation (infrequent, hard stools).

Constipation from peripheral neuropathy usually happens gradually over time and can worsen with each chemo treatment. It's usually mild but, in severe cases, can lead to cramping, nausea, bloating, pressure, or even intestinal blockage. You may already be dealing with constipation because of the effects of other medicines you're taking. Pain medication and nausea-blocking medicines can also cause constipation. That's why prevention is the key. If you're receiving treatment with a vinca alkaloid, your doctor and nurses will ask you if you're having difficulty with constipation and advise you of the steps you need to take to keep your bowels moving.

Here are suggestions that can help prevent or relieve constipation:

- Eat high-fiber foods, including fruits, vegetables, and cereals. High-fiber foods create bulk, which stimulates your colon to move things along.

- Stool softeners and laxatives help the stool in your colon hold on to more water and stimulate the colon.

- Staying well hydrated helps. Drink two to three liters of nonalcoholic fluids daily.

- Physical activity stimulates metabolism and the natural movement of your intestines.

Be sure to talk to your doctor or nurse if you aren't moving your bowels as frequently as you normally do. They can recommend medications and foods that will help relieve your symptoms. See Chapter 6 ("Coping with Other Digestion Changes") for more information and suggestions to prevent and relieve constipation.

PERIPHERAL NEUROPATHY AND HEARING LOSS

Your ability to hear depends on sound waves and vibrations. Your ear is an amazing and delicate instrument that can catch a sound wave and direct it to your eardrum. There the sound is changed to vibrations, which are transmitted to a spiral, fluid-filled organ in your inner ear called the *cochlea*. The vibrations cause tiny hairs (that line the cochlea) to move, creating nerve signals that your brain interprets as sound. If those tiny hairs or nerves are damaged, you can develop hearing loss.

Some chemotherapy drugs, such as cisplatin (Platinol) and high doses of carboplatin (Paraplatin), can damage the sensory hair cells in the inner ear and their connecting nerve fibers. Sound waves can still move through to the inner ear, but they can no longer be changed into nerve impulses. So the sound doesn't reach the brain. This usually affects high-frequency sounds, such as birds chirping, high voices, or music in the higher registers.

Sometimes damage to the inner ear can be experienced as "ringing" in your ears or in your head. The medical term for this is *tinnitus*. The ringing is often experienced as a high-pitched whine or roar, and it can occur in one or both ears. Both of these problems tend to be cumulative over time and are more likely with higher doses of chemotherapy drugs.

Your doctor may order an evaluation by an *audiologist* (a hearing specialist) before your treatment starts if you're already having problems with hearing loss or tinnitus. You may be retested later if you notice a worsening of this problem. Be sure to let your doctor know if hearing loss or ringing develops at any time. If your hearing changes significantly, your physician may change the dose of your chemo or change to a different treatment plan.

You should also follow these recommendations to protect your hearing:

- Minimize any other causes that can decrease your hearing. See your doctor promptly for signs of ear infection, "swimmer's ear," or earwax buildup.

- Avoid other medications that can cause hearing loss, if possible. These include certain antibiotics (such as gentamycin), certain diuretics (such as furosemide [Lasix]), high-dose aspirin, some anti-inflammatory drugs, and some medications to correct high iron levels.

- Protect your ears by avoiding or limiting your exposure to loud noises. Be careful of stereo headphones that are too loud or concerts where the music is blasting. Avoid other sources of loud noise when possible, such as leaf blowers, power saws, lawn mowers, and loud motorcycle or boat engines. Protect your hearing by wearing earplugs when necessary.

- Try to stay well hydrated (drink lots of fluids) after your treatment. That will help eliminate the chemo from your body sooner and lessen the exposure of these delicate cochlea hairs to possible damage.

CHEMO BRAIN

We all have a little trouble concentrating or remembering things sometimes. It might happen when we're particularly stressed or tired. We forget where we put our keys, or we miss an appointment because we didn't write it down. There are times when it's hard to concentrate when having a conversation or while reading a book.

Some people report that they experience more difficulty with memory or concentration during the period when they're receiving chemotherapy. They may refer to it as "chemo brain," "chemo fog," or "brain fog." A common medical term used for this phenomenon is *mild cognitive impairment.*

The symptoms most often reported during this time are difficulty concentrating, short-term memory loss, difficulty performing multiple tasks at the same time (multitasking), and difficulty with language, such as remembering common words. Some people describe it as trying to think through a fog.

Many people don't develop any memory or other cognitive problems from chemotherapy. For people who do experience chemo brain, the effects are usually subtle and not noticeable to others. And they usually resolve over a short period of time.

Causes and Contributing Factors

It's not known exactly what causes chemo brain. The impact of chemo drugs on brain cells is not well understood. But researchers and physicians are becoming more interested and are conducting more studies to examine possible causes. One theory is that chemotherapy can cause direct toxic injury to brain cells. Another theory is that cancer or chemotherapy triggers the body's inflammatory or immune response, which causes injury to brain cells. Researchers are also looking at ways to protect the brain during treatment to prevent cognitive problems.

The effect of chemotherapy on brain cells is not the only reason you might be having this problem. Other factors, such as changes in your diet or sleep patterns, pain, stress, anemia, or the effects of other medications may also contribute to difficulties with memory, concentration, and multitasking. Let your doctor or nurse know how your treatment is affecting you can be eliminated so that some of the factors that can make chemo brain worse and you can get more suggestions to help you get through this time.

Low red-blood-cell count (anemia). After several treatments, you may develop anemia, because chemotherapy can slow down red-blood-cell production in your bone marrow. When your red-blood-cell count is low, there aren't enough of these cells to carry oxygen to your brain and the rest of your body. Your brain is particularly vulnerable to low levels of oxygen in the blood. When this happens, your brain can't function normally. Your doctor may prescribe medication that will help your bone marrow produce more red cells sooner so that you have more energy—physically and mentally.

Poor nutrition. When you're receiving chemotherapy, your body needs good nutrition to help your normal cells recover and to give you energy. Nutrition also plays a key role in the brain's function. For example, low levels of iron, vitamin B, and folic acid can reduce your ability to pay attention, and that can affect your memory. So it's particularly important that you eat a healthy diet. While you're in treatment, you may experience nausea, queasiness, taste changes, or loss of appetite. Maintaining good nutrition is a real challenge. See chapter 7 ("Maintaining Good Nutrition") for more information about your body's nutritional needs during cancer treatment and for recommendations for a healthy diet. You can also talk to a nutritionist who specializes in helping those going through chemo for more advice about how to get the nutrition you need to feed your mind as well as your body.

Fatigue and lack of sleep. Both are very common during this time. When you're tired from lack of sleep, you're more likely to be forgetful and to have difficulty concentrating. Although fatigue is inevitable at times, there are things you can do to minimize its effects and to improve your ability to cope. Talk to your doctor if you're having difficulty sleeping. Many things can make it difficult to get to sleep or stay asleep. For more information about fatigue, including specific suggestions about how to relieve your fatigue and improve your sleep, see chapter 8 ("Coping with Fatigue").

Pain. Many people with cancer don't have pain. But if you're experiencing pain, it can affect how clearly you think. It may be difficult to concentrate on anything other than the pain. Also, pain is often more noticeable at night, when it can interfere with your sleep. If you don't sleep well, you'll probably have difficulty concentrating and remembering things the next day.

Talk with your doctor and nurses about pain management. Report any pain you're experiencing, especially pain that interferes with your sleep. They can adjust your medication so that it works better for you. This can help improve your sleep and thus your memory and concentration.

Other medications. You may be taking many different drugs to prevent side effects of cancer treatments or to relieve pain. Some of these medications can affect your memory and concentration. For example, some pain and nausea-blocking medications can make you drowsy and less alert. Other medications (like steroids) can make you feel anxious and make it difficult to concentrate or to sleep. Also, hormone-blocking drugs can contribute to memory loss.

Sometimes side effects lessen after you've taken a medication for a while. For instance, the drowsiness associated with pain medication may decrease over time. If you're troubled by the side effects of any of your medications, talk to your physician. It's often possible to switch to a different prescription that would have fewer side effects that affect your alertness.

Stress. Feelings of worry and anxiety are inevitable when dealing with cancer and its treatment. You may have concerns about many aspects of your life: family, job, finances, and the future. Even though worry and anxiety are normal in this situation, these feelings can make you distracted and forgetful. Also, worries often seem worse at night, so they can make it difficult for you to sleep.

There are many relaxation and stress-reduction techniques that may help you get through high-stress times. Simply concentrating on your breathing can help. Take slow, deep breaths to release tension and relax your body and your mind. Progressive muscle relaxation (PMR) teaches your whole body to relax through a step-by-step system of tightening and then relaxing groups of muscles. See chapter 14 ("Relaxation and Stress Reduction") for more information and instructions for these and other relaxation techniques. You may also try massage or healing touch, yoga, meditation, or pleasant distractions such as listening to music. Strategies that direct your mind away from worries and support your body to release tension can decrease stress and refresh your mind.

Depression. We all have feelings of depression at times. These feelings usually come and go, alternating with more positive feelings. When you're feeling depressed, it can be difficult for you to concentrate and remember things. If you've had problems with depression in the past, the stress and anxiety of dealing with cancer and its treatments can be particularly difficult.

There are several things you can do to improve your mood when you feel down. Talk to a good friend who's understanding and supportive. Watch a funny movie or a TV show that makes you laugh out loud. Take a walk or exercise aerobically. When you're active, you generate *endorphins*: the "feel-good" chemicals your body produces that relieve pain, anxiety, and depression.

If you find that you feel depressed most of the time, let your doctor know so that you can get help during this time. A referral to a counselor (social worker, psychologist) who can provide extra support may be helpful for you. Medications may also be helpful, because they can relieve depression, anxiety, and sleep problems. A referral to a psychiatrist, especially one who specializes in helping people who are facing medical problems, can also provide the help you need. For more information about depression and other emotional issues you may be experiencing, see chapter 13 ("Mind and Body").

Coping with Chemo Brain

Coping with cancer and cancer treatment is difficult enough. When you also have to cope with short-term memory loss or difficulty with concentration, it could affect your relationships, work, studies, and so many aspects of your daily life. Fortunately, there are many ways to help you cope with the temporary effects of chemo brain.

PHYSICAL HEALTH

In the previous section, we discussed some of the contributing factors that may affect your memory or concentration. Eating well and getting enough rest and sleep are important ways to keep your brain healthy and functioning at its best. Here are several more things you can do to support your brain physically.

Exercise. Your brain doesn't work well if it doesn't get enough oxygen. Regular physical activity increases circulation and the flow of oxygen to the brain. It also improves sleep, reduces fatigue, and improves mood. Even when receiving chemotherapy, you can walk, cycle, or swim. See chapter 8 ("Coping with Fatigue") for more information and suggestions about exercise during treatment.

Reduce your intake of alcohol. Drinking alcohol can impair the functioning of your brain by affecting concentration and making you drowsy. Alcohol can also impair your sleep.

Reduce your use of stimulants. Caffeine and nicotine can make you anxious. Anxiety makes it difficult to concentrate when you're awake and prevents you from sleeping when you want to rest.

Support your senses. If your vision or hearing is compromised, your brain isn't taking in clear information. Wear your glasses or hearing aids if you need them. Work with good lighting, eliminate distracting noises in your environment, and try to minimize distractions when you need to concentrate.

MENTAL HEALTH

Reducing distracting worries and anxiety, and using relaxation techniques are good ways to manage your stress and support your mental functioning. Here are other ways to support the functioning of your mind and help you cope with chemo brain:

Keep your mind active. Exercise your brain by reading, actively listening to music, writing in a journal, or doing memory puzzles (crosswords, jumbles, sudoku). Learning something new is a great way to exercise your mind. Take a class to learn a language, try a craft, or expand your knowledge about an interest of yours (history, boating, politics, and so on).

Support your memory. You can help your memory function more effectively by keeping reminder notes, lists, and a daily calendar. A pocket organizer can be a good tool to use for these tasks. You can keep track of appointments, schedules, to-do lists and shopping lists, birthdays and anniversaries, and phone numbers and addresses. With this kind of support, you'll feel more confident that you aren't forgetting something important.

Establish and stick to routines. This will help you to remember your regular activities and tasks. Also, if you put objects in the same place each time, you'll know where to find them. So have a designated spot for keys, bills, and other commonly misplaced items.

Simplify your life. Break big tasks into small, manageable tasks. For example, pay a few bills weekly instead of saving them all until the end of the month. Reduce unnecessary activities. Set up automatic bill payments for your phone, cable, electricity, and other utilities to save you time and effort. Shop online, when possible, to save yourself time and the energy needed for driving, parking, shopping, and carrying packages.

Avoid multitasking. Try not to do multiple things at once. If you focus on one thing at a time, you can better concentrate on what you're doing.

Reduce or eliminate background noise. Music, TV, and radio can be distracting when you're trying to concentrate on a task or conversation. Without these distractions, you'll be better able to focus.

Ask for repetition. Feel free to ask people to repeat what they've said when it's something you particularly want to remember. The repetition will help you recall it later. Also, if possible, make a note of the information right away.

Be patient with yourself. Don't push yourself too hard. If you can't focus on your work or tasks, give yourself a break. Rent a movie, take a walk, or take a nap. Return to the task when you're rested and focused.

Keep things in perspective. Don't worry about the small stuff. If you're experiencing problems with memory or concentration, it's probably much more noticeable to you than it is to others. You can explain to others that you need more rest, less stress, and their patience. When your treatment is over, you'll slowly regain your clarity and focus.

SOCIAL SUPPORT

Getting support and help from other people is another good way to cope with chemo brain.

Get support. Sometimes talking to others who are also experiencing chemo brain can be beneficial. It can be helpful to know that you're not the only person struggling with this problem. Many people are happy to share their coping strategies. You can join a cancer support group to connect with other people who are having similar experiences. There may also be people in your family, faith community, or neighborhood who've "been there" and know what you're going through. Also, the American Cancer Society may be able to connect you to a cancer survivor who has had a similar experience.

Ask for help, and be specific. Other people probably aren't aware of the cognitive difficulties you're experiencing. This is especially true if you're experiencing these symptoms intermittently: some days your brain works fine, and other days you feel as if you're in a fog. It's important to communicate how you feel and what others can do that would be most helpful to you. People are often glad to help but don't know how. If you tell them specifically what you want, you're more likely to get the help you need.

For instance, one way someone can help you while you're having memory problems is to go with you to your medical appointments. Your support person can take notes so that you're free to listen and ask questions. Your friend can also remind you to ask the doctor about a concern that you may have forgotten. Another way someone can help you is with insurance and medical paperwork. You may find it helpful to have someone handle bills, receipts, authorizations, forms, and refunds. That can be overwhelming to many, whether or not they have concentration problems!

IN CONCLUSION

Peripheral neuropathy and chemo brain may never be problems associated with your treatment. If you do get one or the other, hopefully it won't be more than a nuisance that resolves over time as your nerve endings, brain cells, or both heal. While you do have symptoms, there are many ways to minimize the effects and cope with them.

Chapter 11

Sexuality

Any health problem can strongly affect your emotions. Coping with cancer and the stress of cancer-fighting treatments can make you feel overwhelmed. You may be worried or even angry about your diagnosis. You may feel pressured by the decisions you're being asked to make about your treatment, or fearful about whether you'll survive. If you're recovering from recent surgery, you may still feel some pain and exhaustion. You may be adjusting to changes in your body from the illness or from surgery. If you've lost a part of your body (visible or not), you may still be grieving.

If you're in a relationship, your partner might be going through many of these same feelings of worry, depression, anger, and grief. These stresses can disrupt the balance of the relationship. Your need for contact, acceptance, and physical comfort may be even greater now, yet your partner may hold back. Your partner may feel overwhelmed or hesitate to initiate physical contact for fear of harming you or adding to your stress.

If sexual contact was something you valued and enjoyed before your illness, your feelings probably haven't changed. But now you may have questions about how the illness or its treatment may affect your ability to be sexual. You may not feel comfortable asking your doctor or nurse about these concerns; questions about sex may seem unimportant or inappropriate in comparison to the life-and-death issues that are being dealt with. But information about how cancer or cancer treatment affects you sexually is important to your recovery. When is it safe to have sexual intercourse? How will the medicine you're taking affect you sexually? Will you still be able to have an erection or experience orgasm?

Many myths about sex and cancer cause people much unnecessary anguish. Your mother may have complained that she was no longer interested in sex after her hysterectomy. Will that be true for you as well? You may worry that sexual activity may be harmful or painful after surgery, especially if the surgery involved the reproductive organs or breasts. You may worry that the cancer was caused by sexual activity. Some people fear that they can give cancer to their partners by intimate contact. These myths are not only untrue but also damaging. If either you or your partner believes them, you risk losing the closeness and enjoyment of a sexual relationship.

One way of dispelling a myth is to ask your doctor or nurse about your concerns and get the facts clarified. If you do ask, you'll learn that hormonal changes, menopausal symptoms, hysterectomy, or breast surgery don't necessarily mean the end of sexual enjoyment. Prostate or bowel surgery doesn't necessarily mean that a man can no longer have an erection or experience orgasm. Sex is not harmful to the person recovering from cancer, nor will it spread the disease. It is possible to conceive a child during chemotherapy, so it's important to use effective birth control at this time.

The following sections will help you understand some of the basic facts regarding cancer and sexuality.

CHANGES IN SENSATION

All sensations, whether or not they're sexual, depend on the nerves carrying information to and from your brain via the spinal cord. Nerves to the sexual organs can be damaged from the pressure of a tumor on the nerves, the spinal cord, or the brain. These nerves can also be damaged as a result of the surgery done to remove the cancer. Fortunately, today's improved nerve-sparing surgical techniques are less damaging to the organs and nerves that affect sexual functioning.

Medications can also affect your nerves. Some chemotherapy medicines can cause numbness in the nerves, which can affect your fingers and hands, as well as your legs and feet. The numbness can lessen your sense of touch. Other medicines that you may be taking to relieve pain or nausea can diminish sexual responsiveness.

CHANGES IN HORMONES

A hormone is a chemical substance produced by one organ that's carried by the blood and affects other organs. For instance, insulin is a hormone produced by your pancreas. It's carried by the blood to other cells in your body, allowing them to absorb or use sugar.

The sex hormones are responsible for the development of secondary sex characteristics and fertility in both men and women. These hormones are produced in the mature reproductive organs (ovaries in women, testes in men). Small amounts of both estrogen and testosterone are also produced in the adrenal glands, located near the kidneys. Although both sexes produce estrogen (the female sex hormone) and testosterone (the male sex hormone), men produce a great deal more testosterone, and women produce a great deal more estrogen.

At puberty, testosterone causes the male genitals to enlarge and the testes to produce sperm. It also stimulates the development of other characteristics, such as male distribution of body hair, voice changes, body build, and sex drive. Although the level of testosterone may slow down as a man ages, a man can continue to produce testosterone and sperm for his entire life.

In women, estrogen is responsible for the increase in size of the reproductive organs (uterus, cervix, vagina, ovaries), female distribution of body hair, body build, and the development of breasts. Since most of a woman's estrogen is produced in the ovaries, when these secretions slow down during menopause, the drop in estrogen level causes a number of physical changes. Without enough estrogen, the vaginal lining is thinner, drier, and less elastic. Also, the supply of blood to the vagina decreases. The cervix (the opening to the uterus) produces less mucous, and less lubrication is produced during sexual arousal. The loss of estrogen can also cause hot flashes, mood swings, and fatigue.

The hormonal changes of menopause normally develop slowly over a number of years. But if the ovaries have been removed by surgery or stop functioning because of the effects of chemotherapy, the result can be a sudden drop in a woman's estrogen level and more rapid menopause. Characteristic hot flashes can be more frequent and severe than with normal menopause. Some women can take hormone pills, which replace estrogen (as well as other hormones), to relieve many menopausal symptoms. But some kinds of cancer can also be stimulated to grow more rapidly in the presence of estrogen or progesterone, so hormone replacement therapy (HRT) may not be possible.

Men can also be affected by hormonal changes. If surgery, medication, or chemotherapy reduces the production of testosterone, a man may experience some loss of sexual drive. Over time he'll notice changes in hair distribution as well as changes in muscle and fat distribution. As with women, some cancers in men grow more rapidly in the presence of sex hormones, and in these cases doctors may prescribe anti-androgen hormones to turn off testosterone production. Some new, nonsteroidal anti-androgen hormones are effective in lowering testosterone levels while having fewer detrimental effects on a man's sexual drive or ability to have an erection.

GETTING INFORMATION

If surgery or other cancer treatment will cause changes in your ability to function sexually, even temporarily, you need to know about it ahead of time. Physicians (especially surgeons) recognize their obligation to provide you with enough information to understand the reasons for, risks of, and alternatives to their recommended treatments. If your regular visits to the oncology office or clinic are too brief to allow you to discuss your concerns, you and your partner can make a "talking appointment" with your physician. Take a list of questions that are important to you: How will your ability to enjoy sex be affected? Will treatment affect your sexual desire? Will your ability to have an erection or orgasm be affected? Does the doctor expect that the problem will be temporary, reversible, or permanent? When will you and your partner be able to resume your normal sexual activities?

If your physician can't answer your questions, she may refer you to a specialist for further evaluation. A *urologist* is a specialist in the urinary tract of both sexes and the genital and reproductive functioning of men. A *neurologist* is a specialist in diseases involving the nerves and sensations of your body, including the brain and spinal cord. A *gynecologist* is a specialist in the reproductive functioning of women. Any of these physician specialists might be helpful in addressing your concerns.

In some cases, short-term sexual counseling with your partner can give both of you the opportunity to explore feelings, fears, and needs around sexuality. A specialist may also be a resource for learning about other sexual positions or means of stimulation that will maximize your enjoyment during this time. You can find a qualified sexuality therapist through the American Association of Sexuality Educators, Counselors, and Therapists (AASECT). Support groups can also be helpful, especially if the group includes others who've had the same kind of cancer or the same kind of cancer-fighting treatment. You may get some ideas about how other couples deal with the changes in their sexual lives. The American Cancer Society (ACS) publishes two in-depth booklets on sexuality and cancer: one for men and one for women. They're available for free by calling 1-800-ACS-2345, or online at *www.cancer.org*.

THINGS THAT CAN HELP MEN

If a man loses his ability to get or keep an erection because of surgery, reduced testosterone levels, or drugs, there are several options to consider. Prescription oral medications may improve partial erections, although these medications aren't safe for men with certain medical conditions, such as heart disease. Nonsurgical vacuum devices can also improve partial erections and are safe for most men. A hollow plastic tube is placed over the penis, and a small pump is used to create a vacuum, which draws blood into and enlarges the penis. Urethral suppositories and penile injections are other nonsurgical treatments that can be used to create an erection. Surgical techniques are also available to try to restore erections, using penile implants. One type of implant has semirigid rods that keep the penis partially erect at all times. It can be bent slightly for concealment. Another type of implant uses inflatable rods. This implant inflates or deflates with a small pump implanted in the scrotum and a small reservoir of sterile fluid implanted in the abdomen. Squeezing the pump produces an erection by pumping sterile fluid from the reservoir.

THINGS THAT CAN HELP WOMEN

For women, the lack of estrogen can make intercourse painful because of the changes in their vaginal lining and lack of natural lubrication. If intercourse causes irritation, use a water-based lubricant such as K-Y Jelly or Astroglide. Some women can use an estrogen or testosterone cream, tablet, or intravaginal ring to counteract the effects of menopause on their vaginal tissue.

If intercourse is painful or difficult due to tight vaginal muscles, Kegel exercises may help you to learn how to relax them. To do these exercises, tighten your pelvic muscles as if you're stopping your stream of urine. Hold for a count of three and relax. Repeat ten times. Do these exercises at least twice a day, when your bladder is empty. A vaginal dilator may also help you learn to relax your pelvic muscles during intercourse. After pelvic radiation, a vaginal dilator may be needed to help stretch out a tight vagina or to prevent scar tissue from forming and causing a tight vagina. A dilator is a plastic or rubber tube that comes in different sizes. A woman gently inserts it into her vagina and tightens and relaxes her muscles until it's fully inserted. The dilator is then left in place for a period of time (about fifteen minutes) several times a week. Over time, if needed, she can progress to larger dilators so that the vagina is slowly stretched enough to allow intercourse.

CHANGES IN BODY IMAGE

Your body image is the picture you have in your mind about your physical self. That picture helps form a sense of who you are. A positive body image allows you to feel whole, acceptable, and lovable. When that picture changes, there's necessarily a period of adjustment until you can adapt to the new sense of who you are.

People react very differently to physical changes. Some women experience a hysterectomy as a relief. They're rid of their menstrual periods and no longer have to worry about birth control. Other women may grieve for the loss of the uterus and menstrual periods, because this loss signifies the end of the potential for having children and the disappearance of a function that's tied to their femininity and sexuality. Even if a woman's uterus contained cancer cells and the surgery to remove it may have been lifesaving, she can still feel the hysterectomy as a loss and a change in body image that takes time to integrate.

Body Image and Cancer Therapies

Just having cancer can be tremendously disturbing to your body image, especially if you've always felt strong and healthy. Surgery or other treatments that alter your body either temporarily or permanently can be even more traumatic, and when these changes are noticeable or disfiguring, the natural process of grieving lasts longer. Dealing with cancer treatment can profoundly affect your self-esteem, confidence, and sexuality. If you dread looking at your scar after breast surgery or at your stoma (the opening on your abdomen where part of the bowel protrudes) after bowel surgery, you're likely to worry about how your partner will react or how these changes will affect the way you share your body during intimate sexual contact.

The effects of chemotherapy can greatly alter your body image as well. Hair loss is perhaps the greatest assault to your picture of yourself, but pallor and weight changes can also make you feel self-conscious about your body. A temporary intravenous line that's implanted in or emerges from your chest or arm may feel foreign and obtrusive.

Fatigue, nausea, or the sedating effects of pain and antinausea medication can prevent you from feeling sexual in your usual way. Your body may not feel as if it belongs to you anymore, but, rather, to the doctors and nurses. It's no wonder that many people are reluctant to reestablish sexual contact while feeling this way.

Adjusting to Body Image Changes

The way you react to the physical changes caused by cancer and cancer therapies is personal. The amount of time it takes to adjust to these changes varies from person to person and from couple to couple. There's no right timetable, nor is there an ideal way that couples should deal with these problems. Some people are comfortable sharing the entire experience with their partners, having them present during doctors' visits, dressing changes, and any educational or supportive contact with other health care professionals. In that way, they learn together and are able to reinforce the information for each other. Partners can ask their own questions and get clarification when needed. Other people want more independence or privacy, preferring to absorb the information at their own pace and share the information with their partners as they feel more comfortable over time.

Some people are more comfortable if they camouflage changes in their bodies when they're intimate. There are soft, fiber-filled "night bras" that can be worn under nightgowns to camouflage a missing breast. To cover a stoma and collection bag after a colostomy, some people wear a soft cotton cummerbund. Other couples feel closer to their partners if they can share themselves as freely as they did before surgery and grow used to the changes together over time. Either choice is fine; it's a matter of doing what feels comfortable for you.

For some people, reconstructive surgery makes a big difference in how they feel about their bodies—all the physical adjustments seem easier. Other people feel that additional surgery would be traumatic, especially at a time when they may still be facing months of chemotherapy. Reconstruction may be something they'd consider after treatment is over, if at all. In any case, feeling whole, attractive, and sexual is not dependent on reconstructive surgery.

RESUMING SEXUAL ACTIVITY

Even when the doctor assures you that it's physically safe to resume sexual relations, you may not feel ready. You may need more time to heal, physically and emotionally. Or you may want to engage only in gentle sex play or sex that doesn't involve intercourse. Good communication is more important now than ever if you're to find a way to share sexual intimacy that's satisfying to both of you. Go slowly. Let your partner know how you're feeling and what's comfortable for you. Your partner may be reluctant to initiate sexual activity at all out of fear of harming you, so your encouragement and re-assurance are important.

If you take pain medication or a muscle relaxant, be sure to allow at least a half hour for it to work. Be aware that medications can also make you sleepy or limit your arousal. A warm bath or soothing massage is another way to feel more comfortable before sex. Soft music, candles, and aromatherapy can help you relax and get in the mood.

You may find that certain positions are more comfortable for you or that you need to use a pillow to protect a tender incision or support a part of your body for comfort. Let yourself experiment with ways of pleasuring each other that allow you to feel close without pushing your physical or emotional limits.

Chemotherapy may be present in your body fluids for a few days after each treatment. If you're sexually active at this time, it's important to use a condom to protect your partner from any chemo that may be in your semen or vaginal secretions. Your doctor can give you more information about this based on the specific chemotherapy drugs you're receiving.

BIRTH CONTROL DURING TREATMENT

Many types of chemotherapy will decrease your fertility. However, it's still possible to conceive a child during this time. This is true even if a woman's menstrual periods have stopped as a result of treatment.

Conceiving a child during treatment may not be safe for the baby or for a woman with cancer. Some chemo drugs may damage eggs or sperm. If conception occurs with a damaged egg or sperm, it can result in a miscarriage, a stillbirth, or birth defects. Even if conception occurs with a normal egg and sperm in a woman with cancer, her cancer treatment can be risky to the baby, especially early in the pregnancy.

If a pregnant woman needs chemotherapy, her oncologist will work with the obstetrician about how to protect the unborn baby during her treatment.

So a sexually active couple should use one or more effective birth control methods to prevent pregnancy during cancer treatment. Talk to your doctor about which methods are safe for you. For example, birth control pills contain hormones, which can stimulate the growth of hormone-sensitive tumors, such as some breast cancers. And intra-uterine devices (IUDs) have an increased risk of infection, which can be a problem during chemo. The use of a condom and spermicide are generally safe, effective choices during cancer treatment.

IN CONCLUSION

Your sexuality is not located in any specific organ, nor is it limited to any specific activity. It's much more than that. Your sexuality is a reflection of how you feel about yourself as a man or a woman. It depends, in part, on your acceptance and appreciation of your body as a source of pleasure to you and your partner. Your sexuality is shaped by your memories and experiences, and it changes throughout your life. Because of your illness, you may need to change some of the ways you express your sexuality, but your need to give and receive some form of loving sexual touch won't change.

Your ability to establish and maintain a sexual connection with someone contributes to the quality of your life. Even though, in times of stress or illness, having sex may be the last thing on your mind, the need to love and care for another and to be loved and cared for in return is always there. Sexual contact is something that's not only possible during your illness and treatments—it can also be a source of comfort, reassurance, passion, and joy.

Chapter 12

Fertility

Many couples who hope to have children in the future are concerned about how cancer or cancer-fighting treatments will affect their fertility. This is an important issue to discuss with your doctor. Whether or not it's possible to preserve your ability to have children depends on a number of things: the kind of cancer you have; your sex and age; and the amount, duration, and types of chemotherapy drugs you receive. In general, every attempt will be made to preserve your fertility without jeopardizing the effectiveness of your treatment. For some people, the effects on fertility may not be ascertained until after all the treatments are over and the body has a chance to recover.

GET INFORMATION

If protecting your fertility is important to you, you need to plan ahead before beginning cancer treatment since just one treatment can dramatically affect your fertility. Talk to your doctor right away and find out if you're at risk of infertility because of the kind of cancer you have or from the planned treatments.

Ask your oncologist if there are other effective treatments for your cancer that may have a lower risk of infertility. Then talk to an experienced fertility doctor and find out what your options are before you begin cancer treatment. Your oncologist can refer you to a reproductive endocrinologist, urologist, or gynecologist who specializes in infertility in people with cancer. You may need to go to a university medical center to find this type of specialist.

A variety of reproductive options is currently available, and new techniques are being developed and tested. Men and women who want to preserve their fertility may have the option of freezing and saving sperm, eggs, or embryos. Protective shielding may be used during treatments for men and women receiving radiation to the pelvic area. There are also surgical options that may be appropriate for women with gynecologic cancer.

If you want to pursue one or more options, remember: time is of the essence. For women, pursuing these options may take several weeks, which may delay your treatment for that long. Your oncologist can tell you what the time frame is. In many cases, cancer-fighting treatments may not start right away, because you need several weeks to recover from surgery and to have additional diagnostic tests. Once you have all the information, you can get the process started. Your oncologist and your fertility doctor can work together to coordinate your treatments.

FERTILITY: THE BASICS

Fertility depends on whether a man's sperm attaches to a woman's egg, and whether they attach to the woman's uterus and grow and develop into a baby. Each sperm and each egg contain genetic material. When they combine to create a unique individual, this genetic material gives the child the attributes of both parents. Here's an overview of how this happens naturally along with some useful terminology.

The Life of a Sperm

At puberty, the pituitary gland in the male brain starts sending hormone signals to both *testes* (in the scrotum) to start sperm production. After that, throughout his life, a man can continuously produce sperm.

Sperm cells look different from other cells. They have a head, neck, body, and tail. The head is the part that can attach to a woman's egg (*ovum*), and the tail allows the sperm to move quickly (like swimming) through a woman's cervix, uterus, and fallopian tubes. The ability of sperm to move is called *motility*.

Newly created sperm move from each testis into a winding tube (*epididymis*) on the top of each testis. This is where they mature. Then they move into a straight tube (*vas deferens*), where they remain until they're released.

When a man is sexually stimulated, sperm are released into a long tube (*urethra*) where they combine with fluids from the *seminal vesicles* and *prostate gland* to make *seminal fluid* (also called *semen*). Muscles at the base of the penis contract, and sperm and seminal fluid are expelled through the penis during *ejaculation*. Normally, about four hundred million sperm are expelled during each ejaculation.

Male fertility depends on the quantity and quality of sperm ejaculated and their motility. If there aren't enough sperm, they don't have a normal shape, they have poor motility, or they aren't able to attach to an egg, the chances of conception are limited.

The Life of an Egg

Women are born with a limited number of eggs (*ova*) in their *ovaries*. They start to mature at puberty when hormones from the pituitary gland in the female brain start sending signals to the ovaries.

Unlike sperm, which are continuously produced and released in large amounts, usually only one egg (*ovum*) is produced and released during a woman's monthly cycle. This is how it happens: Each month, hormone signals stimulate the ovaries to grow and mature a number of *follicles* (fluid sacs). Inside these follicles are eggs. Soon, one follicle and its egg begin to grow bigger than the rest. When the egg matures, it's expelled from its follicle and the ovary. This is called *ovulation*. The egg then travels into a long, narrow tube (*fallopian tube*) connected to the *uterus* (womb). The expelled egg remains capable of being fertilized for about two days.

While the follicle and egg are growing and maturing, hormone signals sent from the ovaries are stimulating the lining of the uterus to thicken and prepare for pregnancy. If pregnancy doesn't occur, the egg and uterine lining pass out of the body (called *menstruation*), and a new monthly cycle begins.

Female fertility depends on a woman's monthly menstrual cycle. A complex system of hormone signals regulates this cycle and the changes in the reproductive organs. Fertility ends with menopause, when these hormone signals stop.

Fertilization

When semen is ejaculated into the vagina during sexual intercourse, sperm swim from the vagina into the uterus through the opening called the *cervix* and up into the fallopian tubes. If they meet the egg in one of the fallopian tubes, they try to attach to the egg. If one is successful, *fertilization* occurs. The fertilized egg journeys through the fallopian tube into the uterus. When it comes into contact with the thickened lining of the uterus, it attaches and accesses the uterine blood supply for nutrition and oxygen. This process is called *implantation*.

If the pregnancy proceeds normally, the fertilized egg (*embryo*) develops into a *fetus*. And about forty weeks later, a baby is born.

REPRODUCTIVE EFFECTS OF TREATMENT FOR MEN

Some types of cancer, such as testicular cancer and Hodgkin's lymphoma, can affect fertility by reducing the number of sperm or by damaging sperm so that they don't swim well.

Cancer treatment can also affect fertility. This is because it can kill rapidly dividing cells such as those found in the part of the testes that constantly produces sperm. So when a man receives chemotherapy (or radiation therapy to or near his testes), sperm-producing cells are damaged or killed, and sperm production decreases or stops. Any sperm that are produced during this period are likely to be damaged or have poor motility, decreasing their ability to reach the egg inside a woman's body or to produce a healthy child.

Infertility from cancer treatment may be temporary or permanent. If sperm production resumes after treatment, it usually will happen within the first two years.

Some chemotherapy drugs are more damaging to male fertility than others. It may be possible for your oncologist to substitute a different drug that will be less damaging to the sperm-producing cells of the testes. As a general rule for chemotherapy, the larger the dose and the longer the period of treatment, the more likely it is that your fertility will be affected.

REPRODUCTIVE OPTIONS FOR MEN BEFORE OR DURING TREATMENT

If your treatment may cause infertility, you may have one or more of the following options to preserve your ability to father children. Before you begin cancer treatment, talk to your oncologist and a fertility specialist about which ones are appropriate for you.

Sperm Banking

A good option for many men is to save their sperm in a sperm bank. This enables men to preserve viable sperm that can be used many years later. Even if you aren't sure that you want to have children in the future or don't currently have a partner, it may be a good idea to save your sperm before treatment so that you have that choice later in life. It may not be an option if the cancer itself has caused abnormal sperm or decreased sperm motility.

To save sperm, you provide one or more sperm samples before you begin treatment. You can go to a sperm bank to provide samples, or collect samples at home and take or mail them to a sperm bank. The samples are then frozen and can be stored for an indefinite period of time.

When you want to conceive a child, your sperm sample can be thawed and used to fertilize a woman's egg in the lab in a process called *in vitro fertilization* (*IVF*). If the sample has a large number of sperm with good motility, it can be placed in your partner's uterus in hopes that one of your sperm will fertilize her egg and create a pregnancy. This is called *intrauterine insemination* (*IUI*). It's a quick and easy procedure done in a doctor's office. The thawed sperm are prepared and inserted in her uterus with a thin tube during the most fertile part of her monthly cycle.

Even if the sample has only a few sperm, *intracytoplasmic sperm injection* (*ICSI*) can be used to fertilize an egg. ICSI is a specialized type of IVF where a tiny hollow needle picks up a single sperm and then injects it through the egg's surface to the inside (cytoplasm) of the egg. Then this fertilized egg can be implanted into the woman's uterus.

Testicular Sperm Extraction

If you want to save sperm but can't provide a sperm sample or don't have mature sperm in your semen, testicular sperm extraction may be an option. A doctor can perform this outpatient procedure using a needle to obtain tiny pieces of testicular tissue, which are examined for sperm. If found, the sperm can then be frozen and stored in a sperm bank for future use. Or the sperm can be used immediately to fertilize an egg with ICSI. The embryo (fertilized egg) can be implanted in your partner or frozen and stored for later implantation. This procedure can be done either before you start cancer treatment or after you finish treatment.

Radiation Shielding

For men who receive radiation treatment to their pelvic area, radiation shielding is an easy way to help preserve their fertility. Depending on the location of the cancer and the radiation field, special shielding may be used during treatments to reduce the amount of radiation to one or both of the testes. This can help reduce the risk of testicular damage and infertility. Radiation shielding does not provide protection from chemotherapy, because chemo goes through your bloodstream and reaches every part of your body.

In the Future

Research into new ways of protecting and restoring men's fertility is ongoing. New procedures and medications that are considered experimental now, like all advances in medicine, may someday become the standard of care.

One example of a procedure that may be available in the future is *testicular tissue freezing*. This is an outpatient procedure performed before cancer treatment. A needle biopsy is used to obtain a sample of testicular tissue. The tissue is then frozen and stored for transplantation back into the man's body after treatment is completed. The hope is that the tissue will produce sperm after it's transplanted back into the body.

REPRODUCTIVE EFFECTS OF TREATMENT FOR WOMEN

Chemotherapy or pelvic radiation can affect the ovaries so that there are fewer available eggs. Damage to a woman's limited egg supply can prevent healthy eggs from maturing and being available for ovulation and fertilization. This can cause infertility.

Also as a result of chemo (or radiation to the pelvic area), a woman's ovaries may stop producing the hormones that are essential for fertility. This can cause her menstrual periods to stop during treatment. When this happens, it causes early menopause and can result in infertility. In some cases, women's periods resume after treatment, and their fertility returns. This can happen as long as four years after treatment. But even if a woman's periods return after treatment, her egg supply could have been damaged, so she may still be infertile. Or she may regain fertility temporarily but then go through menopause and become permanently infertile much earlier than normal.

Radiation treatment to the pelvic area can also damage the uterus or cervix, causing scarring and damaged blood vessels and making it difficult to carry a baby to full term.

As with men, the kind of chemotherapy, dose, and length of treatment are all factors that will influence whether the ovaries will

continue to produce mature eggs and secrete the hormones necessary for conception. For women receiving radiation therapy, the risk
of infertility depends on their age, amount of radiation, and site of
radiation.

REPRODUCTIVE OPTIONS FOR WOMEN BEFORE OR DURING TREATMENT

If you're a woman facing potential loss of fertility from cancer treatment, you may have the following options for preserving your ability
to have children. Talk to your oncologist and a fertility specialist
about which options are appropriate and safe for you.

Embryo Freezing

Embryo freezing is the most common and successful way for a
woman to preserve her fertility. This process involves removing mature
eggs from a woman's ovaries, fertilizing them with sperm from her
partner or a donor, and freezing and storing the embryos (fertilized
eggs) for a future pregnancy.

There's a better chance of a successful pregnancy if multiple
eggs are retrieved and fertilized and multiple embryos are stored, so
hormones are usually administered to stimulate a woman's ovaries
to develop multiple mature eggs. When the eggs are mature, the
woman undergoes an outpatient procedure to retrieve the eggs. With
the assistance of an ultrasound machine to "see" the ovarian follicles
(fluid sacs), a needle is inserted to remove the mature eggs from the
ovaries. The eggs are then fertilized with sperm in the lab using IVF
or ICSI, and the embryos are frozen and stored. After treatment,
when the woman is ready to get pregnant, the embryos are thawed
and implanted in her uterus using IUI.

Although embryo freezing can be very successful, the process
requires two to six weeks to stimulate the ovaries to produce multiple
eggs. This can delay your cancer treatment. In addition, the hormonal
stimulation usually used for this process (and for egg freezing) may

not be safe for women with some types of breast, uterine, or ovarian cancers. The hormones you would receive to stimulate egg production will increase estrogen to a level much higher than normal, and this can cause estrogen-dependent cancers to grow or spread.

If you have an estrogen-dependent cancer, there are other options that allow egg collection without hormonal stimulation. But only one or sometimes two eggs can be collected during a woman's natural ovulation cycle without hormonal stimulation. Other techniques have been developed recently to prevent estrogen from stimulating the cancer to grow or spread during this time. One option uses the anti-estrogen drug *tamoxifen* instead of hormones to stimulate the development of mature eggs. Tamoxifen also blocks estrogen from affecting breast tissue and encouraging cancer cell growth. Another option uses an *aromatase inhibitor* (such as letrozole) in combination with hormonal stimulation. Letrozole keeps the level of estrogen in the body close to natural levels during this process.

Egg Freezing

Egg freezing involves retrieving mature eggs with the same procedure as embryo freezing, but the eggs are frozen without being fertilized by sperm. This option may be appropriate for you if you don't have a partner to contribute sperm and don't want to use donor sperm. The rate of successful pregnancies is not as high as it is for embryo freezing, because unfertilized eggs are more likely to be damaged during the freezing or thawing process. However, new techniques for freezing and fertilizing eggs are increasing the number of successful pregnancies.

As with embryo freezing, hormones are usually given to stimulate the ovaries to mature multiple eggs. The eggs are then surgically retrieved, frozen, and stored for a later pregnancy. Once thawed, eggs are fertilized with sperm in the lab and the embryos are implanted in the uterus to try to create a pregnancy.

As with embryo freezing, this process can take several weeks and can have the same risk of delaying the start of cancer treatment.

Radiation Shielding

Women who receive radiation therapy to their pelvic area may be able to have special shielding placed, during treatments, to protect their reproductive organs. If this can be done, it may reduce your risk of infertility from radiation damage. This shielding does not provide any protection from chemotherapy because chemo goes throughout your body.

Ovarian Transposition

Ovarian transposition is an outpatient surgical procedure that reduces the risk of radiation damage to the ovaries and the risk of infertility. A woman who will receive radiation therapy to her pelvic area may be able to have this procedure before starting her treatments. During the procedure, a surgeon moves the ovaries away from the radiation "field" or target area. The procedure needs to be done close to the start of radiation therapy, because the ovaries tend to fall back into place over time.

Radical Trachelectomy

Radical trachelectomy is a surgical option for women with early cervical cancer. During the woman's cancer surgery, the surgeon removes most or all of the cervix but leaves the uterus and ovaries in place. With this procedure, it may still be possible to carry a pregnancy, although a suture (surgical stitches) may be needed to hold the uterus closed during the pregnancy to prevent a miscarriage or premature birth. Specialized medical care and monitoring would be needed during the pregnancy.

In the Future

Protecting a woman's fertility is the focus of many research efforts. Two options that are currently experimental but may be available for women in the future are described here.

Ovarian tissue freezing. *Ovarian tissue freezing* is a surgical approach currently being studied. A surgeon removes all or part of one or both ovaries prior to the start of cancer treatment. Tissue from the ovary is then frozen and stored for later transplantation back into the woman's body after her treatment is completed and she's ready to try to get pregnant. If successful, the transplanted tissue produces hormones and mature eggs. The eggs are retrieved using a needle biopsy and fertilized in vitro. This may be an option if you don't have the time necessary for hormonal stimulation and embryo or egg freezing.

Ovarian suppression. *Ovarian suppression* is currently being studied as a way to prevent chemotherapy and pelvic radiation from causing infertility. A monthly hormone injection is given during the period when you're getting chemo (or radiation). This hormone stops the ovaries from functioning and causes temporary menopause. While the ovaries are shut down, chemo and radiation may be less damaging to the ovaries and eggs. Then, when treatments are finished and the hormones are stopped, the hope is that the ovaries will start working and the eggs will be able to mature normally.

EVALUATING YOUR FERTILITY AFTER TREATMENT

After the completion of treatment and before trying to conceive, men should have lab tests to check their hormone levels, and a semen analysis to check the amount and quality of the sperm they're producing. Women should have fertility testing that includes lab tests to check their hormone levels and an ultrasound to check their reproductive organs and egg supply. Also, if there has been damage to a woman's uterus or cervix, she should discuss this with an obstetrician before trying to get pregnant to ensure that she'll be able to carry a pregnancy. Be sure to check with your oncologist about when it's safe for you to begin planning a pregnancy.

REPRODUCTIVE OPTIONS
AFTER TREATMENT

Men and women have a variety of options for having a child after cancer treatment.

Options for Men

The possibilities for men are natural conception, assisted reproduction, and donor sperm.

Natural conception. After treatment most men start making at least some sperm. This usually happens sometime during the first two years. If enough mature sperm are produced and they have good motility, a man may be able to father a child naturally, through sexual intercourse.

Assisted reproduction. If a man saved sperm in a sperm bank, it can be used to fertilize his partner's eggs with IVF, and the eggs can be implanted in his partner's uterus to create a pregnancy. Or the sperm can be placed in his partner's uterus with IUI. If the man didn't save sperm, a fertility doctor may be able to find and extract individual sperm from his testes. This procedure, called testicular sperm extraction, was described earlier in this chapter.

Donor sperm. Men who don't produce sperm after cancer treatment have the option of using donor sperm. This is an easy, relatively inexpensive, and highly successful way for a man who is infertile after cancer treatment to become a father. The donor sperm samples are tested for sexually transmitted diseases (STDs). Donors also go through a detailed screening so that you can select a donor whose characteristics closely match your own. The sperm sample selected is placed in your partner's uterus with IUI.

Options for Women

The possibilities for women are natural pregnancy, assisted reproduction, donor eggs and embryos, and surrogacy.

Natural pregnancy. For some women, chemo doesn't affect their fertility. They continue to produce healthy, mature eggs and can get pregnant naturally. Some women temporarily lose their fertility, but their ability to produce healthy, mature eggs returns after cancer treatment. This usually happens within the first four years. These women may also be able to get pregnant naturally, without medical intervention.

Assisted reproduction. If a woman saved embryos prior to her treatment, she can have them implanted in her uterus to create a pregnancy. If she saved eggs, IVF can be used to create embryos that will be implanted in her uterus to try to create a pregnancy.

Donor eggs and embryos. If a woman doesn't have healthy eggs but does have a healthy uterus, she has the option of using donor eggs from another woman. The eggs could come from an anonymous donor or someone the woman knows, such as a friend or family member. A donor goes through a careful screening process to check for genetic diseases, STDs, and any other health or emotional issues. IVF is used to fertilize the donor's eggs with sperm from the woman's partner. The woman is given hormones to prepare her uterus for the donor eggs. Then the embryos are transferred to her uterus to create a pregnancy. The hormones used in this procedure may not be safe for a woman with hormone-sensitive cancer.

Similarly, donor embryos can be used to try to create a pregnancy in a woman with a healthy uterus. Donor embryos usually come from other couples who have frozen embryos during infertility treatment and who don't want to have more children. If early menopause is the cause of a woman's infertility, a fertility specialist may also be able to help her to get pregnant using donor eggs or embryos.

Surrogacy. Women who don't have a healthy uterus or whose health would be at risk from a pregnancy have the option of having another woman carry the pregnancy and give birth to the baby. This is called *surrogacy*. A surrogate can be implanted with embryos from the parent couple. Or the surrogate can be artificially inseminated with sperm from the male partner. Another option is for the surrogate to be impregnated with donor eggs or embryos.

Surrogacy laws vary in different states and in different countries, so it's important to have an attorney who understands the laws where you and the surrogate live. Also, it's important for the surrogate to have physical and mental health evaluations to ensure that she's healthy and stable. All parties need to understand the legal limits and obligations of a surrogacy contract.

Adoption

Adoption is also an option for someone who wants to become a parent after cancer treatment. You can adopt a child in most states through a public or private agency or independently, without the assistance of an agency. Or you can use a private agency to adopt a child from a foreign country.

If you use an adoption agency, it's best to choose one that works with cancer survivors and is familiar with their unique issues. Before beginning the process, you'll probably need to provide a letter from your doctor about your health.

In the past, most adoptions were "closed," which means that the adoptive parents and the birth parents never had contact with each other after the adoption. This is still true for most foreign adoptions. But many adoptions within the United States are now "open." This means that the adoptive parents and birth parents exchange information and, if desired, maintain contact with each other and the child.

COSTS

The cost of infertility treatments will vary. The more complex interventions requiring lab tests, medications, scans, and surgical procedures will be more expensive. Sperm banking and storage will cost much less. Check with your insurance company to see whether treatments to help with infertility caused by cancer treatment are a covered benefit. Some policies may cover some or all of the costs.

Before you make a decision, check out the fertility programs that are available in your area. You can compare their costs as well as their success rates. Your oncologist might be a good resource to find the physician or clinic that has the most experience.

IN CONCLUSION

Becoming a parent for the first time (or adding another child to your family) may be an important milestone for you—a dream you have for the future. But when you are faced with a cancer diagnosis, you may wonder if having a child will still be an option once your treatments are completed. Whether or not it's possible to preserve or resume your reproductive capacity depends on many factors: the kind of cancer you have, the kind of treatments you need, your age, and so on. That's why it's important to get information from your oncologist and from fertility specialists. There are many resources available to help you understand your options and give you support along the way. Whether you get to become a parent with or without medical assistance, or with a donor, an adoption, or a surrogate, there may be a way to achieve this goal.

For additional information about reproductive options, research studies, insurance coverage, and financial assistance, you can contact Fertile Hope, a national nonprofit organization that provides reproductive information and support to cancer patients and survivors whose medical treatments can cause infertility. You can access their website at www.fertilehope.org or call them toll-free at 1-888-994-HOPE.

The American Cancer Society is also a good source of information about infertility and reproductive options for cancer survivors. Their website is www.cancer.org, and their phone number is 1-800-ACS-2345.

Chapter 13

Mind and Body
by Burton A. Presberg, MD

I listen to people tell stories about their lives and cancer. They talk about their families, jobs, and living situations. They tell how cancer has profoundly changed their lives. Cancer affects much more than bodies. Life itself is suddenly different in almost every way. The preceding chapters detailed many of the physical aspects of cancer and its treatment; this chapter focuses on the mental and emotional aspects. This chapter is about you, the human being who happens to have gotten this disease.

The chapter is divided into four sections. The first is about emotions. You may be experiencing a whole range of feelings; this first section is about understanding and accepting them. The next section addresses the connection between mind and body: what we know and don't know in this controversial area. The third section focuses on methods to help you cope, live, and feel better. These include counseling, support groups, religion and spirituality, and other complementary therapies. The final section provides some hints for finding the path that's right for you.

Dealing with cancer is difficult and challenging. It can feel awful and unfair. Nevertheless, you can use your strengths and the support of others to cope to the best of your ability. The obstacles on the journey are many; hopefully this chapter will provide you with some strategies to maneuver through them.

THE EMOTIONAL IMPACT OF CANCER

Receiving a cancer diagnosis is extremely traumatic. This is true regardless of the type of cancer, its stage, and whether the diagnosis was expected or unexpected. A variety of emotions may emerge, and these feelings may stay constant or may change repeatedly. You may feel like screaming or crying, or you may feel engulfed in a fog. The shock may alternate with numbness, in which you may feel nothing or even "forget" that you have cancer. Then cancer suddenly jumps back into your awareness and you feel scared, angry, and overwhelmed. You may recognize your emotions as being similar to an experience of losing a loved one or receiving other devastating news. This back-and-forth shows the struggle your mind is having with accepting unwanted news. Minds work this way. You're not going crazy, even though it may feel like it at times.

Initial shock is often followed by a period of activity. This is the time to learn more about the illness and treatment options. You gather your strength, identify your supports, and make necessary work and home arrangements. This is a period of rearranging priorities, determining what's really important to you, and perhaps learning to appreciate little things more. This may well be the period that you're in now, as you read this book.

Fear, anger, and sadness are some of the many emotions you may be feeling. These responses may be very difficult to accept, particularly if you're used to feeling in control. In addition to the fact that your body isn't acting as you would like, your emotions are running out of control. Treatment and its side effects, particularly fatigue, sleeplessness, and nausea, add to these mood swings.

It's very important to understand that all of this is normal. Simply allowing yourself to have all of these feelings is a crucial step. Of course, everyone differs in degree of comfort in expressing emotions, but, as much as possible, try to let it out. You may wish to do it by yourself, with friends and loved ones, or with a therapist or support group.

The necessity of thinking positively is a myth. The whole spectrum of emotions, from negative to positive, is unavoidable and necessary. Not letting yourself feel your actual feelings or getting upset at yourself for being angry or sad can backfire, causing you to feel even worse than you did before. On the other hand, a good cry or yell is often relieving and healing. Feelings provide us with vital information. Denying them or keeping them inside may in fact be the unhealthy choice.

Your mind may continue to fight the truth at times, but eventually reality sets in. The cancer exists and however much you dream and wish for its sudden disappearance, the struggle continues—at least for now. Accepting reality doesn't mean being passive. Instead it means doing everything you can do to help yourself while simultaneously learning to live with what can't be changed. You'll learn to live your life with cancer, perhaps in better ways than you ever expected. A shift often takes place—a shift from feeling like a victim, from wondering "why me," to feeling that living the best you can with your illness is a challenge and a motivation.

Sadness Is Okay, Depression Is Not

Having cancer is undeniably difficult, physically and emotionally. Sadness is expected; it's normal and inevitable. The feeling of sadness is often called depression, but clinical depression (also called major depression) is entirely different. *Clinical depression* is a reversible illness. It extends beyond normal sadness to cloud every aspect of the sufferer's existence. In a physically healthy person, problems with sleeping, eating, and maintaining energy point toward a diagnosis of clinical depression. In a person with cancer, difficulties in these areas are almost universal. Therefore they can't be used to determine whether a person has depression.

Distinguishing normal sadness from clinical depression in a person who has cancer depends on psychological symptoms. People with cancer feel sad but still feel that they're good people. A person with clinical depression has a poor self-image. A sad person can still enjoy activities and relationships; someone with depression loses the ability to feel pleasure and often withdraws from family and friends. Sad people maintain a balanced view of the world and feel capable of doing things to help themselves. People with clinical depression often feel that the entire world is hopeless and that they're entirely helpless and unable to change any aspect of the situation. While a sad person may think about death, a person with depression dwells on death and often has suicidal thoughts.

Identifying clinical depression is important because it's treatable. Treatment includes counseling and, often, an antidepressant medication such as Lexapro, Paxil, Zoloft, Cymbalta, Desyrel, or Wellbutrin. Medications often take a number of weeks to work, but over time, mood and outlook usually improve significantly. Side effects, particularly with the newer antidepressants, are generally minimal. Antidepressants work by raising the level of certain chemicals in the brain. These chemicals (called *neurotransmitters*) stabilize mood and control anxiety. The goal is to help you feel like yourself, undoubtedly dealing with a difficult situation, but still the same person underneath. Antidepressants don't block feelings of sadness or take away your feelings, nor do they cause dependence.

If you feel that you may be suffering from depression, please speak with your doctor. You or your doctor may wish to consult with a mental health professional about counseling. Consultation with a psychiatrist about medication is also a possibility, though any physician can prescribe antidepressants.

Family and Friends

This is a time in your life when, more than ever, you need the support of family and friends. You need concrete physical support, such as help with medical paperwork, transportation, and housework. You also need emotional support: someone to listen and provide a shoulder to cry on.

Asking for support isn't always easy. You may not want to bother anyone, or you may worry about having your privacy invaded by an army of helpers. It's particularly hard for those of us who are used to giving aid rather than being aided. It's a slow, step-by-step process to get comfortable asking for help. A useful way to look at this is that, in most cases, others want to be there for you. This allows them to feel useful and needed during a difficult time for everyone. Allowing others to be supportive can really be your way of helping *them*—allowing them in rather than shutting them out.

Be patient with yourself and those around you. Be clear with others about what you need and what you don't need. Don't expect others to be able to read your mind. Having cancer can significantly change relationships, roles, and responsibilities. During treatment you may not be able to pull your own weight at home or at work, and it's going to take time and effort to reassign responsibilities. Resentments may come up, as well as old fights you thought were long behind you. Open discussion and communication have never been more important.

MIND AND BODY: WHAT'S THE CONNECTION?

The relationship between the mind and the body has been debated throughout human history. Our ancestors had no doubt of the connection, and ancient rituals were designed to heal mind and body together. The rise of medical science in the twentieth century led to the opposite viewpoint: the view that mind and body are split and unrelated. Medical science has focused on cells, chemicals, CAT scans, and other measurable physical realities. Recently the pendulum has begun to swing back, and many are preaching the unity of mind and body. Whom should you believe?

The Appeal and Limitations of Mind-Body Unity

At the basic level there's no doubt that mind and body are inextricably connected. Blushing from embarrassment or feeling "butterflies in your stomach" from nervousness reminds you of this reality. Fear causes goose bumps. Research has clearly demonstrated the connection between a type A personality and heart disease. But what does this mean for the person with cancer? The truth is somewhere in the middle. Mind and body undoubtedly interact and work together. But the details of the connection aren't clear and are often overstated. This in itself can be dangerous, leading to guilt over having "caused" your own illness and feeling extraordinary pressure to heal yourself.

Certainly, living a happy, stress-free life while keeping a positive attitude is admirable, but for most of us, it's much more easily said than done. The problem is that you may feel pressured to make changes in your life that are unrealistic and unattainable. The mind may account for some changes in the body, but you certainly can't be expected to heal your cancer simply by thinking it away. The mind controls the body to some extent, but certainly not completely.

Unfortunately, cancer is a powerful biological illness. The mind-body advocates are tapping into a universal human wish: the desire to have control of one's own life and destiny. It's no wonder that people flock to any approach that promises a cure. The downside comes when the mind-body approaches don't succeed in curing.

Dangers: Guilt, Responsibility, and Quackery

The mind-body approaches may lead to feelings of guilt or responsibility. You may feel guilty when you're unable to will away your cancer. Oversubscribing to mind-body views can put too much responsibility on your already burdened shoulders, weight you may not be willing to bear. It's one thing to work together with your doctor to do what can be done; it's another to feel that all of a sudden, you have to change everything about the way you think, feel, and relate to the world.

Quackery is a significant danger. Unfortunately, many people prey on those who are willing to consider anything that can provide a sense of hope and control. Investigate alternative methods carefully and run, don't walk, away from anyone who promises a cure. The risk is losing a lot of money, or worse, physical endangerment from untested methodologies that conflict with or interact adversely with other medical care. While physicians vary in their views of these alternative therapies, it is crucial to talk with yours to find out if there are specific risks to your health.

You Did Not Ask for Cancer

This is a crucial point. Even if you have lung cancer clearly related to smoking, you did not intend to get the disease. It's also crucial to understand that despite suggestions that depression, anxiety, stress, or personality can cause cancer, there's no good scientific evidence to prove this. We all have anxiety and stress in our lives, so it's easy for someone who gets cancer to imagine that it was caused by these things. Some of the calmest, happiest people get cancer, and some of the most depressed, stressed-out people never get cancer. Blaming yourself for your illness is unnecessary, unproductive, and most importantly, unfair.

It's understandable that you would try to find a reason for your cancer. People want events to make sense. We want there to be an explanation for why things happen. Unfortunately, with cancer there is often no satisfactory explanation. Sometimes things just happen with no rhyme or reason. Justice and fairness do not always prevail.

Where All This Leaves You

The bottom line is this: mind and body work both together and separately. The connection is real but not absolute. Addressing where your mind, thoughts, and emotions are during this experience is important for its own sake. Your mind creates your perception of reality and your experience of your life. Respect the profound importance of this, but don't take it too far.

Practically speaking, this means doing what feels right to you. It means accepting the unknown and realizing that there are no guarantees. Take care of both your mind and your body as best you can. If visualizing white blood cells fighting cancer feels right to you, do it. If it doesn't, spend your time in other ways.

The challenge is being open to new ideas and approaches yet skeptical at the same time. The key is clarity of purpose. If used to improve well-being and quality of life, a number of mind-body approaches can be very useful. If, on the other hand, the goal is to cure cancer, trouble may arise.

HELP ALONG THE WAY

There's plenty of help available. Struggling with cancer, its treatment, and your own feelings is not something you have to do alone. The approaches are numerous and varied. This section introduces some of the possible avenues you may wish to pursue to help you cope and live your life with cancer.

Individual Counseling

Talking to a therapist is an option to consider. You're going through a lot right now, both physically and emotionally. Talking with family and friends can be very helpful. Still, it's very different to talk to an objective outsider. A therapist or counselor doesn't have personal ties to you, so the relationship exists entirely for you. You may feel the need to comfort and soothe your loved ones and may not wish to subject them to your sad, angry, or other difficult feelings. With a therapist, you express it all. Simply voicing your feelings to another person can be comforting and freeing.

It's important to find a therapist who has experience in working with people with cancer. Your medical system may have designated support people, or your doctors or nurses may have practitioners they've referred people to before. The type of therapist isn't as important as finding someone you feel comfortable talking to. You'll want to seek out an MD (psychiatrist) if medication issues are likely to be involved, but otherwise, a psychologist with a Ph.D., a master's-level counselor, and a social worker are all possibilities.

Make sure that you and your therapist are clear on the goals and process of therapy. Sessions may be scheduled on an as-needed basis or more regularly, such as once a week or once every two weeks. Clarify the type of therapy you want and need. Therapy can focus on bolstering your existing coping mechanisms (supportive psychotherapy), looking at personality issues and conflicts (exploratory psychotherapy), changing thought processes (cognitive psychotherapy), or providing stress management and relaxation exercises (behavior therapy). Therapy may include combinations of these therapies, as well.

Other therapy options involve couples or family work. Talking things out with your partner or family members in the presence of a trained facilitator can be very helpful. During this time, old tensions may worsen or new questions may arise. What should you tell your children? Who is going to cook when you're feeling ill?

Flexibility is the key in counseling; your therapy issues and needs may be very different at different points in your illness. At times you may not feel well enough to talk; other times you may wish to meet more frequently. Choose a therapist who is flexible and willing to accommodate your changing needs.

Support Groups

Cancer support groups are becoming increasingly popular. It's no wonder—who better to talk to about cancer than others facing the same challenge? At the deepest level, the only people who understand what having cancer is like are others with cancer.

Just as with individual therapy, there are different kinds of support groups. Groups may be for people with cancer, family members of those with cancer, or both together. They may be for people with a specific type or stage of cancer or for people undergoing a specific type of treatment. Groups may be time limited (meet for a certain duration, such as eight or ten sessions) or ongoing, with no set ending date. They may meet weekly, every other week, or monthly. They may or may not be led by a professional. They may focus on supportive sharing, teaching by invited guests, visualization and relaxation exercises, or a combination of these formats.

To find the best group for you, start with your health care team. Groups may be offered on site, or referrals can be given to local groups. Other sources of information on cancer support groups are your local American Cancer Society office, the ACS website (www .cancer.org), and the National Cancer Institute's Cancer Information Service (1-800-4-CANCER).

A support group may not feel helpful immediately. It's often difficult to hear about the hard times of others, and it may be difficult to share your feelings in front of strangers. You may get annoyed at or dislike other group members. After all, all kinds of people get cancer. Give yourself time to get used to the group and to the people. I recommend attending four to six sessions before deciding to leave a group. After that, if you aren't happy with the group, it's possible that it simply doesn't fit your needs, or even that groups are not for you. As with everything else, trust your intuition and feelings; proceed on the course that feels best for you. For many, this path includes a support group of others who have cancer.

Religion and Spirituality

Religion and spirituality can be powerful tools for coping with illness. This may involve traditional religious structure and institutions or your own individual beliefs and practices. Either way, this can be a profound source of comfort and understanding. Spiritual and religious views serve as a guidepost and anchor in times of stress and difficulty. At a time when you feel overwhelmed, religious and spiritual ideas help give an understanding of the unknown and a sense of the meaning of life and death. Spiritual traditions can provide a feeling that the world's much larger than your own individual problems. In addition, they offer an understanding of the purpose of your life as a human being.

Religious institutions also provide a sense of community. This helps you feel less alone as you face your illness. Considerable practical help is available, such as with meals, transportation, and child care. Certainly your openness to religion depends on your background and past experiences. Still, many find that their cancer experience has given them an opportunity to begin exploration of spiritual issues. Many hospitals have chaplaincy services with personnel experienced in dealing with cancer-related issues.

Other Complementary Therapies

Mind-body approaches are numerous and are known by many names, including "alternative," "holistic," and "unconventional." I'll use the term *complementary therapies*. This stresses the fact that they should be used along with conventional medical therapy, instead of in its place.

Physical approaches include exercise, yoga, massage, acupuncture, tai chi, chi gong, and other forms of bodywork. These are wonderful for keeping your body physically active. There's a lot that Western medicine doesn't understand about how the body works as a whole. The Eastern theory is that the body has channels of energy or life force (chi) that are opened and redirected through these various techniques. Many have been used for thousands of years.

Psychological methods include relaxation, visualization, meditation, hypnosis, counseling, and support groups. Relaxation, visualization, meditation, and hypnosis are all techniques to quiet and focus the mind. The benefits include an increased awareness and appreciation of the present moment and a feeling of connection and unity with other people and the world around you. Several of these techniques are described in chapter 14 ("Relaxation and Stress Reduction").

Spiritual avenues include prayer and spiritual counseling. Prayer, both by and for you, is getting a lot of attention these days. Some studies say it helps. It certainly can't hurt.

Creative-arts therapies include art, dance, drama, music, and writing therapies. Whether you're a beginner or expert in one or more of these techniques, a creative outlet for dealing with your feelings can be quite illuminating and useful. For many, feelings emerge more easily via a creative outlet than in traditional talking therapies.

I worked with a woman with breast cancer who struggled with the issue of complementary therapies. Friends and family members told her to meditate, visualize, and get acupuncture. Many of her friends said they had heard stories of "miracle cures" and urged her to try anything, including going to Mexico to try an untested medical treatment. She carefully talked through her options and decided against going to Mexico. Her family and friends were in the United States, and she had developed a trusting relationship with her oncologist. Over time she decided to try a class on mindfulness meditation and found that it helped her feel relaxed and at peace with herself. She realized that meditation alone wouldn't cure her cancer, but simply feeling better seemed like an important and attainable goal. She remains in remission and is working and spending time with her family. She knows the future is uncertain but says that she feels she's learning to be more comfortable living with that uncertainty. After all, she says, the future is uncertain for everyone, even those without cancer.

FINDING YOUR OWN PATH

Even with the support of your family, friends, and health care team, your cancer is a very personal and individual experience. It's a challenge to find your own way to treat and live with illness. Have faith in your feelings, your hunches, and your intuitions. There's a fine balance to strive for: the balance between hope and acceptance. Hope for the best; hope for a cure; hope for the highest quality of life possible. At the same time, accept that there are no guarantees. Unfortunately, modern medicine does not have all the answers. Working with the system and accepting its limitations (as well as your own) isn't easy, but it's crucial for your sense of well-being.

There Is No One Right Way

If there were one answer to cancer, everyone would follow the same recipe. Since there's not, there are confusing choices to be made. Gather all of the support and information that you feel you need. Discuss your choices with your physician and nurse. If certain complementary therapies feel right to you, do them. If not, don't. Be easy on yourself. Sometimes after a diagnosis of cancer, people expect to change their personalities overnight. Eventually changes may occur, but at least at the beginning, it's best to use the coping mechanisms that have helped you get through other difficulties in your life. You may be a person who copes with adversity by researching every bit of information available. If so, dive into the scientific literature. On the other hand, you may be a person who handles difficult situations by pulling back and trusting others to help you make decisions. Either way, do what works for you.

Individual Coping Styles

Many people will have their own ideas about what you should do and how you should feel. Some will want you to keep a stiff upper lip; others will urge you to let it all hang out. The bottom line is that no matter how things are physically, you are still you inside. People have different ways of coping. Some like to read every study on cancer; others leave that up to the doctor. Some meditate, do yoga, and get acupuncture; others watch a movie, listen to music, pray, or work. Be yourself. Look back at the things (and the people) that have helped you get through hard times in the past. Life is full of challenges, and this includes unfairness and illness. As with other challenges, you'll do the best you can.

Laughing and Loving

Laughter may not come easily, but when it does, let it happen. There's some evidence for the physiological benefits of laughter. It certainly can feel good. Humor involves looking at life from a different perspective. Often this can mean taking serious topics such as illness, life, and death and making fun of them in some way. I've had the good fortune of being witness to humor and mirth in some very unlikely and potentially uncomfortable situations. There's no better tension reliever. While it's not always an appropriate option, look for humor when it's available.

Similarly, feelings of love and contentment may be difficult to find in a mind that's filled with lots of other worries. Finding the time and space to live and love in a busy, imperfect, anxiety-filled world is a challenge we all face. We're all searching for meaning in our lives and our experiences. Sometimes meaning and peace are hidden behind what seems to be an insurmountable wall. The way through is not apparent. On second look, though, you may see gaps in the wall, tools to help you break through, or a way around.

One Day at a Time

The only moment any of us lives in is right now. Yesterday is gone; tomorrow may never come. This reality is never clearer than when you're dealing with a serious physical illness. Many have said that they never felt truly alive until they knew, at the deepest level, that they were going to die. Again, the operative word here is challenge. The challenge is to exist fully and love fully in the series of moments that go together to form today. In this way, the truly important things, your real priorities, show themselves to you.

This, of course, is much easier said than done. To live fully, one day at a time, when you're facing a difficult illness, is certainly not easy. To do it, treat your mind and body well. I wish you all the best on your journey.

About the Author

Burton A. Presberg, MD, has a private practice in psychiatry. He is the former director of psychosocial services at the Alta Bates Comprehensive Cancer Center in Berkeley, California. He works closely with patients, families, and health care practitioners in addressing the multitude of biological, psychological, social, and spiritual issues involved in cancer.

Burt received his BA and MD degrees and psychiatric training from Cornell University. He received fellowship training in Consultation/Liaison Psychiatry and served on the faculty of the

Medical College of Virginia in Richmond, Virginia, prior to beginning his position at the Alta Bates Comprehensive Cancer Center.

SUGGESTED READING

The volume of available literature is enormous and can be overwhelming. In keeping with the tone of the chapter, if it feels useful, read it; if not, put it away. Here are my suggestions of a few books that many have found helpful:

Gordon, James S., and Sharon Curtin. 2000. *Comprehensive Cancer Care: Integrating Alternative, Complementary, and Conventional Therapies.* Cambridge, MA: Perseus Publishing. An expert in alternative medicine addresses cancer care.

Holland, Jimmie, and Sheldon Lewis. 2000. *The Human Side of Cancer: Living with Hope, Coping with Uncertainty.* New York: HarperCollins. One of the founders of the study of psychological aspects of cancer (psycho-oncology), Dr. Holland is compassionate and knowledgeable.

Hopko, Derek, and Carl W. Lejeuz. 2007. *A Cancer Patient's Guide to Overcoming Depression and Anxiety: Getting Through Treatment and Getting Back to Your Life.* Oakland, CA: New Harbinger Publications. A self-help workbook that includes helpful worksheets and exercises.

Jampolsky, Jerry. 1983. *Teach Only Love.* New York: Bantam Books. Written by the founder of the Center for Attitudinal Healing, this book offers an inspirational approach to love, acceptance, and healing.

Kabat-Zinn, Jon. 1994. *Wherever You Go, There You Are: Mindfulness Meditation in Everyday Life.* New York: Hyperion. Beautifully written essays on meditation, stress, and living in the moment. Not specifically focused on cancer.

Kushner, Harold S. 1981. *When Bad Things Happen to Good People.* New York: Avon Books. Written by a prominent clergyman struggling to come to terms with his son's illness and death.

Lasater, Judith. 1995. *Relax and Renew: Restful Yoga for Stressful Times.* Berkeley, CA: Rodmell Press. Presents detailed, step-by-step instructions and photographs of restorative yoga techniques.

Lerner, Michael. 1994. *Choices in Healing: Integrating the Best of Conventional and Complementary Approaches to Cancer.* Cambridge, MA: The MIT Press. Excellent, balanced review of complementary therapies by the founder of Commonweal.

Rossman, Martin L. 2003. *Fighting Cancer from Within: How to Use the Power of Your Mind for Healing.* New York: Henry Holt and Company. Written by a pioneer in the use of guided imagery for healing.

Spiegel, David. 1994. *Living Beyond Limits.* New York: Fawcett. A leader in the study of cancer support groups details his sensible approach to coping with cancer.

Weil, Andrew. 1983. *Health and Healing.* Boston: Houghton-Mifflin. A leader in integrative medicine discusses his view of healing. One of a number of excellent books by Dr. Weil.

Chapter 14

Relaxation and Stress Reduction

Any change that requires us to adapt is a stressor. Positive stress, such as getting a new job, getting married, or leaving home for the first time, requires us to adjust to a desired change in our lives. Negative stress, such as family problems, loss of income, or dealing with illness, requires us to adapt to an unwanted challenge.

We experience acute stress when we're facing imminent danger. Our bodies initiate a series of biochemical changes that prepare us to cope quickly and effectively with threats. This is the "fight-or-flight" response, which was so essential to the survival of our primitive ancestors. Today, although there are no saber-toothed tigers in our midst, the heightened awareness, increased strength, and more responsive reflexes produced by our stress response still help us survive many threats. When you veer to avoid a collision on the freeway or notice that your child has run into the street, you can feel how those chemical changes affect your heart, breathing, muscle tension, blood pressure, metabolism, and so on. Not only can such events trigger the fight-or-flight response, even the mental image of one of these events can make your body react in the same way. Therefore, if your mind continuously returns to a traumatic event, your body constantly responds with a chemical reaction that keeps you in that reactive state.

Chronic stress can occur when the sources of stress are unrelenting, or when many less serious stresses accumulate and you're unable to effectively respond to any of them. It produces the same biochemical changes as acute stress. Over a period of time your body's attempt to respond to unrelieved chronic stress can adversely affect every body system, as well as suppress your immune system—making it harder for your body to heal.

You know how much physical and emotional stress you and your family are experiencing since learning about your cancer diagnosis. Your visits with your doctor, diagnostic tests, procedures, surgery, and even learning what you need to learn to get through your treatment are tremendously stressful. In addition, you may find that your mind returns to traumatic events in the past or that you anticipate future events that could be upsetting or painful. You may want to turn off the stress response, but how do you achieve that when feeling overwhelmed with thoughts and feelings, fears and concerns during this time?

Fortunately there are a number of relaxation techniques that can not only help you lower your stress level but also help you reduce its immunity-suppressing effects. Many of these techniques seem so simple and basic that you can't imagine how they could be effective to prevent and relieve the negative effects of stress. How is it possible that just focusing on your breath can help you when your mind is racing and your body is surging with stress hormones? But these practices work. Breathing, muscle relaxation, and imagery techniques, as well as self-hypnosis, can help you relax your body. Mindfulness and observing your thoughts can help you stay centered and feel less overwhelmed. Other techniques can help you deal with specific fears.

Learning these relaxation techniques will require some practice, and it's best to practice before you're in the stressful situation. It helps if you set aside a few minutes once or twice a day to work on it. Eventually it may even be something to look forward to each day, because you'll start to experience the positive effects. In the book *The Three Minute Meditator* (Harp 1996), the author maintains that even a few minutes a day of clearing your mind and focusing on your breath can help the day go more smoothly. Some techniques require that you close your eyes while doing the exercise. But some can be done anytime or anyplace you need to stop the stress response. You can focus and breathe deeply or use visualization while walking, washing dishes, or waiting to see your doctor.

DEEP BREATHING

Deep breathing is an ancient Eastern technique as well as a modern, medically proven adjunct to Western medicine. It oxygenates your blood while releasing muscle tension in your diaphragm. Deep breathing is an excellent way to achieve very rapid relaxation. It will help you feel better in a hurry when you're facing some immediate stress.

If you want to practice deep breathing, try lying down in a comfortable place. Bend your knees and lay one hand on your abdomen and the other on your chest. Breathe lightly through your nose. In this normal breathing pattern, the hand on your chest and the hand on your abdomen will rise and fall together. But in deep breathing, only the hand on your abdomen will rise, while your chest will move very slightly, if at all. By pushing your breath way down into your abdomen, you not only get more air, but you also stretch your diaphragm so that the tense abdominal muscles can start to relax.

Now try it. Breathe deeply so that only the hand on your abdomen rises with the breath. Breathe in slowly through your nose, pushing up the hand, and then exhale through your mouth. Sometimes it feels good to make a whooshing noise as you let go of the breath.

When you feel ready, take another breath. Breathe only when you feel like it. You're taking in a lot more air than usual, so you'll breathe more slowly than usual. If you rush it and breathe faster than you need to, you're going to get too much oxygen, and you may feel a little dizzy. If that happens, just concentrate on slowing your breathing so that you take a breath only when you need to.

Practice the deep-breathing technique until you feel comfortable with it and it feels easy, almost second nature. You should set aside three or four times during the day to work on your breathing. When you've mastered deep breathing while lying down, practice it sitting in a chair, feet flat on the floor, hands resting on your knees. You'll find the practice comes in handy, because it's an effective way of dealing with the tension you may feel while having an IV started or having your blood drawn in the lab.

BREATHING AND IMAGERY

Autogenic breathing combines deep breathing with imagery for extremely effective stress relief. To learn this technique, start by lying down and doing deep breathing for two to three minutes. When you're in a comfortable rhythm and feeling more relaxed, visualize yourself lying on a warm, white beach. Feel the warmth from the sun caress your skin, radiate into your muscles, and finally seep into your bones. Feel the soft, warm breeze touch your body.

Now imagine being covered with warm sand; the weight of the sand feels like a warm, protective hand on your body. Feel the heavy warmth penetrate deep into your muscles, relaxing and purifying your body. The warmth and the heaviness relax your body more and more deeply.

Now listen to the ebb and flow of your breath. Say to yourself "warm" as your breath comes in, and then "heavy" as your breath goes out; "warm" on the in-breath, "heavy" on the out-breath...warm and heavy...warm and heavy. Really try to feel the warmth in your limbs as you say "warm" on the in-breath. Try to visualize the heavy sand holding your body safe and secure as you breathe out.

Stay on the beach as long as you want, letting the autogenic breathing relax and refresh your body. Practice the imagery until the warmth and heaviness are easy to feel. Practicing this technique at home can pay off later, and the imagery can help you to relax even during extended treatments or diagnostic tests.

OTHER RELAXATION IMAGERY

Visualization is a lovely way to take a break, a vacation from stress. You can go anywhere in your mind, creating a retreat of exquisite peace and beauty. The following three "retreats" will give you an idea of the special places you can go without ever leaving your chair. With just a little practice, you can start designing your own special place that has all the elements you need for deep relaxation. If you can create an image that appeals to all of your senses, it will be even more effective. Notice that the retreats described include many details—not just what the place looks like, but what you would hear and feel if you were really there. Let your imagination take you away.

Retreat 1

It's dark and cool as you begin walking on the path leading upward toward the mountain. Early morning stars and the moon guide you along this trail beside a rushing stream. Slowly you climb, step by step, along the flowered path wet with morning dew. The sky lightens into a pale blue. You know this day will be warm. Cardinals, bluebirds, and wrens start to whistle and sing, keeping you company along the path that begins to open into stands of pine and oak. You walk on, feeling strong and happy that you're alive and eager to stand atop the mountain at sunrise. The stream next to the path trickles over a tiny waterfall. You place your hand under it, drinking its clear, cold water. You walk on. Your body feels light and strong as you climb. The first golden rays of sunlight are just peeking out to your left as the trail reaches the edge of a granite knoll. You're at the top now, and the sun breaks behind the mountain range on the horizon, rising quickly, an enormous ball of power greeting you, warming you, lighting you. You sit on a rock, breathe deeply, and inhale the clean, crisp air. In the valley below, you can see rivers of mist flowing. But here the warm, bright sun shines above you, strengthening you as it does the plants and the birds. Here at the top, you feel a sense of peace and relaxation flowing throughout your entire body.

Retreat 2

You awake slowly in your room by the ocean. Darkness envelops you as you put on your beach slippers and pad out to the screen porch, warm cup in hand. You sit in the rocker, quietly rocking back and forth, listening to the roar of the cresting sea. The stars pierce the sky's black blanket. You breathe quietly, deeply, feeling the rolling of the rocker on the wooden floor. Near the shore, long grasses wave gently, matching the movement of the sea. You are safe. The moist air caresses your face. The warm drink soothes. The sky lightens, and the stars disappear. You can see for miles. The sun rises red over the horizon as pelicans glide between the peaks of the soft sea swells. Light glows, bathing you. You continue to breathe deeply, slowly, mirroring the rhythm of the waves as they run up the shore.

Retreat 3

The weeks have been hectic, but you're safe now on the train. You sink deeply into your seat and watch the vast, pale desert slip past the train window. Buttes stand silent and orange above the sagebrush-covered ground. The sun is setting, and the sky flames red and purple. The light fades slowly, but you can still see the mountains cut against the night sky. The low, rocking thunder of the train wheels blankets all other sounds. You feel safe and peaceful as the train rocks gently under you. You sink more deeply into your seat as you hear the clacking wheels. You have no problems to solve, nothing to think about as the train carries you through the desert night. It holds you, rocking gently as it speeds.

Your retreat may be nothing like these. You may conjure up a room from childhood, the breakfast table at your grandmother's house, a Paris café, a sandbar at the bend of a river, a high meadow, or a campground beneath whispering trees. Go there often; use your retreat when you feel anxious and tired, when you're uncomfortable, when you're bored.

MINDFULNESS

When you pay attention (or listen in) to how your mind is working, you realize that it's constantly producing thoughts—thousands of them every day. Most are fleeting and quickly forgotten; some are persistent and memorable. Your thoughts can help you feel optimistic, encouraged, and happy. Or they can take you to scary places full of dread, fear, and worry. Some thoughts serve us by helping us understand and learn from the past or solve problems and plan for the future. Some fill us with fear and keep us from experiencing the fullness of life. But thoughts are not reality, and we have the ability to observe our thoughts without necessarily believing everything they tell us.

During stressful times people often feel overwhelmed by thoughts that make them feel anxiety, fear, dread, sadness, anger, and so on. They may try to deal with these thoughts by attempting to suppress or escape from them. They may use distraction, work, drugs, or other numbing behaviors to drive them from their own minds. Although that may work for a while, painful thoughts inevitably return. But people can feel less overwhelmed if they learn to observe their thoughts without judgment, without running away—without distraction, suppression, or numbing behaviors. They can learn to question the validity of their thoughts, to recognize the benefit or detriment the thoughts bring to their lives, and how to distance themselves from thoughts that are negative and painful.

The first step is to focus on the present moment—not past memories, not future plans or problems. When you do that, it allows you to get some distance from upsetting or painful thoughts, making them less overwhelming. You can start by attending to your breathing, saying the words "breathe in" on inspiration and "breathe out" on expiration. Or you could count your breaths, from one to four, and then repeat the sequence. You don't need to breathe in any particular way. Just pay attention to the flow of air into your nostrils, the rise and fall of your chest or abdomen, and the release of air.

Noticing your breath is an easy way to focus your mind (you're always breathing!), but you can focus on anything in your environment.

You can focus on a sound (the wind in the trees, water running in a fountain), body sensations (walking, knitting, mowing the lawn), or a visual focal point (looking at a candle, watching the movement of clouds). The following instructions will suggest that you return to your breath, but you can return to any point of focus that you choose.

Next pay attention to the thoughts that come up for you. Just observe them without judgment. Don't decide if they're bad or good—just notice them. Your thoughts might be memories, observations about your environment, judging thoughts, or thoughts that explain why things are the way they are. They may be planning thoughts, problem-solving thoughts, or fantasies. Don't try to hold on to any one, and don't try to get rid of the thought either. Just notice your thought as it occurs and let it go without judgment as you return your focus to your breathing. Notice the thought, let it go, and return to your breathing again and again.

Here's an example. You may have a memory thought about a song that you heard on the radio that morning—let it go and return to your breathing. You may have a planning thought about how you will get home from the clinic—let it go and return to your breathing. You may have a worry thought about whether or not the results of your lab work might mean that your chemotherapy will be delayed—let it go and return to your breathing.

Of course, there will be thoughts that seem to snag your attention and take you away from your focus. For instance, that thought about how you'll get home from the clinic can lead to thoughts about your friend who promised to pick you up but who's usually late. Then you remember the time you were stranded outside the movie theater waiting for her for a half hour and missed the beginning of the movie. Then you think of the movie and try to reconstruct the plot. Then you recall that the star of that movie was in rehab for drug addiction. The chain of thoughts and worries takes you away from your focus. When you notice that has happened, pull yourself back to the present, let it go, and refocus on your breathing.

You may notice that one type of thought comes up more frequently. For instance, during this time you may have a lot of worry thoughts or problem-solving thoughts. Or you may notice that some thoughts trigger strong emotions. Some memory thoughts can trigger feelings of comfort, while others can bring up feelings of anger. What role do these thoughts play in your life? Are they helpful or detrimental? For instance, you may have observed that you thought, "I felt nauseated after my first chemo treatment. I guess nothing will work for me." If you believed that, you would be less likely to let the doctor and nurses know about the problem and less likely to get more effective antinausea medications next time. You don't have a choice about what thoughts arise in your mind, but you do have a choice about how you relate to them. Ask yourself how a particular thought serves you. Does it make you feel more capable, more optimistic, more in control? Does it make you feel more distressed or discouraged or weak? You can't eliminate a discouraging thought, but you don't have to believe it or have it direct or limit your life.

This way of observing your thoughts is called *thought defusion* and is used in acceptance and commitment therapy (ACT). You can learn more about it in the book *Get Out of Your Mind and Into Your Life* (Hayes and Smith, 2005). There are many other exercises that can help you become more aware of how your thoughts can relieve your stress or add to your stress. *Leave Your Mind Behind: The Everyday Practice of Finding Stillness Amid Rushing Thoughts* (McKay and Sutker, 2007) is also highly recommended to anyone wanting to learn more about this powerful technique.

PROGRESSIVE MUSCLE RELAXATION

Progressive muscle relaxation (*PMR*) is a technique developed in the 1920s by Dr. Edmund Jacobson. It's based on the theory that a person cannot be both relaxed and anxious at the same time. To calm anxiety, muscles are progressively tightened and released in sequence throughout your entire body.

In the beginning, PMR takes fifteen to twenty minutes for each practice session. But in a few weeks, after you learn it thoroughly, you can tighten groups of muscles simultaneously and reduce the time it takes to achieve relaxation to just a few minutes. When using this technique, avoid tensing muscles or areas of your body that may be painful. If pain is a problem, just read this section to learn the PMR sequences, and then go on to the section, "Relaxation Without Tension." Before you start, read the instructions completely. At first it may help to write the sequence (right fist, left fist, and so on) on a piece of paper so that you can easily refer to it while doing this exercise.

Basic PMR Procedure

Find a comfortable position, either lying down or sitting in a chair. First, tighten your right fist and forearm. Clench as hard as you can for seven seconds. Notice what the tension feels like. Now release your fist and feel the muscles in your forearm relax for twenty seconds. Notice how relaxation feels: heavy, warm, or tingly. Really experience the relaxation in your hand and forearm. Repeat the procedure with your right fist once again, always noticing as you relax and release the tension. Now do the same thing with your left fist and forearm. Tense for seven seconds and relax for twenty. Now do both fists at the same time, tensing for seven seconds and relaxing for twenty. Always notice how relaxation feels in your muscles.

The next step is to tense the muscles in your right arm. Make them as hard as you can for seven seconds and then relax. Do the tensing and relaxing twice with each arm.

As you continue through the exercise, tighten each specific muscle for seven seconds and relax for twenty. And then repeat the same muscle once again. Pay attention to what relaxation feels like in each muscle.

Now focus on your face, the seat of so much tension. Wrinkle up your forehead. Hold it taut, then release.

Now frown and squint your eyes, holding them tightly shut. Release.

Purse your mouth into an "O." Relax and notice what it's like to let go of tension in this area of your face.

Now tighten your jaw, bite hard, and push your tongue against the roof of your mouth. Relax and notice what it feels like to release the tension in your jaw.

Turning to the neck and shoulder area, press your head back against your chair and then relax your head. Roll slowly and gently to the right and then to the left.

Straighten your head and gently let it fall forward. Relax and really feel the release of tension in your neck.

Now hunch your shoulders. Relax and let them droop, feeling the relaxation spread through your neck, throat, and shoulders.

Feel the relaxation move throughout your entire body. Feel the comfort of the heaviness. Now breathe in and fill your lungs completely. Hold your breath and notice the tension. As you exhale, feel all tension leaving your body. Repeat the full breath several times, paying attention to how tension can drain out of your body as you exhale.

Tighten your abdominal muscles, just as if you were preparing to be punched. When you relax, let the tension drain away again. Put your hand on your belly and push it up with a deep breath. As you let go, feel your entire abdomen relax.

Gently arch your back slightly. Be careful not to strain it. Relax again and take another deep breath.

Tighten the muscles in your lower back. Relax and notice how the muscles feel without tension.

Tighten your buttocks and thighs. Flex your thighs by pressing down your heels as hard as you can. Relax and notice what it's like to let go of tension in these big muscles.

Now curl your toes downward, making your calves tense. Relax.

Now pull your toes back toward your face, creating tension in your shins. Relax again. Observe the muscles in your feet and calves. Notice how it feels for them finally to relax.

Just feel the heaviness throughout your lower body as relaxation deepens. Notice the relaxation in your feet, ankles, calves, shins, knees, thighs, and buttocks. Let the relaxation spread to your stomach, lower back, and chest. Let it become deeper and deeper. Experience the relaxation deepening in your shoulders, neck, arms, and hands. Then experience the feeling of looseness and relaxation in your neck, your jaw, and all your facial muscles. Your whole body feels more and more deeply relaxed.

Shorthand PMR Procedure

After you've practiced PMR for several weeks and are aware of the effects of tension and relaxation on specific muscles, you're ready to shorten the process. You can now tighten and relax certain muscle groups simultaneously. Just as you did before, tighten for seven seconds and relax for twenty, but be sure to avoid painful areas or straining. Carefully observe the effects of both the contraction and the relaxation of your muscles. As your muscles loosen, let your whole body grow heavy and still.

Curl your fists. Tighten your biceps and forearms (in a "Charles Atlas" pose). Relax.

Wrinkle up the muscles of your face like a walnut. Frown with your eyes squinted, lips pursed, tongue pressed against the roof of your mouth. And with the same walnut face, hunch your shoulders. Relax.

Breathe deeply into your abdomen as you slightly arch your back. Hold, observe, and relax. Breathe deeply again, pressing out your abdomen. Hold. And then relax.

Now curl your toes while simultaneously tightening your calves, thighs, and buttocks. Relax. Pull your feet and toes back toward your face, tightening your shins. Hold and relax.

Relaxation Without Tension

This exercise involves relaxing your muscles in the same sequence that you learned with PMR. But there's one difference: you don't tighten each muscle. Instead, you notice any tension that may exist in the muscle and then "relax away" the tightness.

Twice a day, practice going through each muscle in the PMR sequence and "relaxing away" any tension you find. Try to make the muscle feel as relaxed as it did right after you let go in the PMR exercise.

Relaxation without tension allows you to scan your body for "hot spots" of tightness. You can relax away tension in the doctor's office or while you're receiving treatments.

AFFIRMATIONS

You can replace frightening thoughts with positive affirmations. An affirmation is a short statement that helps you feel more self-confident, stronger, and less fearful.

Here's a list of affirmations that you may use. Choose a few that you like and memorize them. Or use them for ideas to create unique affirmations of your own.

About Relaxation

- Relaxation floods my body like a healing golden light.
- Each breath brings a flood of healing power to every corner of my body.
- I am filled with peace, calm, and serenity.
- Relaxation, enjoyment, and love are the things that keep me well.
- Taking care of myself keeps me strong.
- Relaxation is the gift I give myself.
- Every time I breathe in, I bring a wave of peace and relaxation. Every time I breathe out, I let go of tension and fear.

To Reduce Fear About Treatments

- I can get through this.

- I can take care of myself.

- I can ask for what I need.

- The people around me (my nurse, my doctor, my family) know how to make sure that I am safe and comfortable.

- Every treatment takes me another step closer to health and recovery.

- Cancer cells are weak, sick, and confused.

- Chemotherapy is a strong ally. It works with my body's natural defenses to wipe out the defective cancer cells.

- I am open to the healing power of the medications.

After Chemotherapy Treatments

- The chemotherapy has done its job. Now it will be washed out of my body, taking with it the dead cancer cells.

- My body's natural defenses are building again and will be ready to protect me again.

- Chemotherapy is like a great crashing wave. It may shake me up for a minute, but now the water has receded, and I am safe again on the shore.

- Chemotherapy is like a torrential downpour, washing away the weak and broken cancer cells, leaving the strong healthy cells glistening in the sun.

- Chemotherapy has been like allied troops coming to a troubled area, routing the enemy and then returning the region to peace, beauty, and health.

IN CONCLUSION

As you look back at the stress reduction exercises described in this chapter, you can see that there are similarities among them. Most start by having you pay attention to your breathing or another point of focus. When you do that, you bring your awareness to the present moment. Then you can use healing imagery, fantasy, or positive affirmations. You can also lower your anxiety in stressful situations by distancing (defusing) from the constant stress-inducing chatter of your thoughts. PMR gives you physical relief in the areas of your body where you may be holding on to stress. Similar kinds of focusing exercises are used in meditation, biofeedback, and pain management. Other activities, such as playing a musical instrument, listening to music, writing in a journal, and being outdoors in nature, also relieve stress.

Try different exercises and see what works for you in different circumstances. You may do breathing and imagery at night to help you sleep and use mindfulness when you're waiting for your doctor. At first it may be difficult to keep your focus or quiet your mind. But just as when you're learning any new skill, it will get easier with some practice. Even in difficult circumstances, you do have the power to calm your mind and find peace and relief from stress.

Chapter 15

Preparing to Start Chemo: A Practical Guide

You've probably been given a lot of information about your treatment plan, chemotherapy, medications, and prevention and management of side effects. You have papers with phone numbers, reports of scans, lab tests, and pathology reports. The nutritionist and social worker probably gave you more information, along with a schedule of classes and support services. So many handouts! So much paper! This can be overwhelming.

Before you start your first treatment, it will probably help to organize some of this information so that it's accessible and useful to you. If you can put your hands on the information you need when you need it, you'll feel better prepared to start chemotherapy and to take care of yourself after your treatments. This chapter will help you with that. As you read over some of the general items in the chapter, it may remind you of other important issues that you need to take care of. Add them to one of the lists. After your first treatment, when the whole experience is more familiar, you may want to add or subtract from the lists to ensure that you remember the things that are important to you.

BEFORE YOU START CHEMO

Getting the information you need, getting organized, and getting ready are all ways you can be better prepared for chemo. You'll feel less stressed, and the preparation will save you time and energy later.

Get Information

Information about your treatment plan and work options will help you plan your schedule at home and at work. Understanding your insurance coverage and disability benefits will help you plan for any changes in your expenses and income.

√ **Understand your treatment plan and schedule.** You and your doctor will decide on a treatment plan. Be sure that you understand how many treatments are planned (if known), how often you'll get chemotherapy, and how long each treatment is likely to last. Find out if you'll need to come for lab tests and other appointments between chemotherapy treatments. Then you can decide the days of the week and times of day that work best for you, and set up your appointments. Although there may be changes in the schedule as you go along, you can at least start to plan your work and family commitments, and arrange for transportation, child care, and so on.

√ **Understand your insurance coverage.** Your doctor's office probably has a financial counselor who deals with the insurance companies and authorizations. This would be a good person to help you clarify your coverage, or you can call your insurance company directly. You need to know what your insurance will cover (treatments, tests, meds, clinic visits, lab tests) and what your financial obligation is (co-pays, deductibles, limits to the coverage). Are you restricted to certain providers (for instance, network doctors and hospitals)? What tests and treatments require prior authorization? If you want to (and are able to) change your medical or drug benefits, the financial counselor could give you some guidance.

√ **Understand your work options.** If you're employed, ask your manager if there are options for working part-time, from home, on "light duty," or on a flexible schedule. Also, find out if you can move your work environment to an area where you'll have less exposure to infection from other workers.

√ **Understand your disability options.** Talk to your human resources department or union representative about your disability benefits. If you take time off, will you have the same job and schedule when you return? Who will do your job while you're gone? If you qualify for disability payments, how much will you get, when will it start, and how long will it last? The Americans with Disabilities Act (ADA) and the Family Medical Leave Act (FMLA) are federal programs that provide some job protection for you or a family member who may need to take time off to help you. When you apply for disability benefits, remember that it may take another few weeks (or longer) after your final chemotherapy treatment for your strength and energy to return. Factor that into your estimate of when you expect to return to work. It's easier if you overestimate the time off you need and come back early if you feel well enough. It's more difficult to try to extend your disability benefits later if you initially underestimated the time off that you need.

Get Organized

Organizing your medical records, information sheets, resources, phone numbers, and schedule will really help. It will make it easier to communicate more effectively (with the doctors, with your family), get help when you need it, and anticipate and prepare for what you'll need.

√ **Make a list of questions for your doctor and nurse.** Appointments with your doctor can sometimes be stressful and rushed, making it difficult to remember and ask all your questions. Keep a little notebook with you so that you can keep track of the questions that occur to you between appointments. Before you see your doctor, consolidate the list so that you use your time efficiently. If you bring someone with you to the appointment, that person can keep track of your list of concerns, take notes, and help you remember the information.

√   **Make a "chemo binder" or folder.** This is the answer to the mountains of paper you're handed at every turn. A simple binder divided into sections will help you easily find important information and prepare for your appointments. The binder could include:

- Phone numbers for doctor, nurse, nutritionist, after-hours assistance, pharmacy, hospital, and so on

- A calendar for your appointments

- A list of your current medications, including dosages and how often you take them

- Chemo information sheets including information about possible side effects

- Copies of lab and test results for your information and to share with other doctors you see

- Information on classes and support groups that you may want to attend

- Community resources, websites, and other resources that may be helpful to you

- Insurance information

- A compact three-hole punch so you can put your documents away immediately

- Notepad or extra paper so that you can keep a list of your questions and take notes

√   **Assess your support system (family and friends).** Once you determine what kind of help you need, talk to your family and friends to determine who's available. Be realistic about their availability and talents and their own obligations. Be specific about what's expected. Do you need a ride to or from the clinic? Someone to keep you company during your treatments? Child care? Shopping? Food preparation? Keep a list of a few people who might be available for unscheduled errands to the pharmacy or to feed your pets if you're delayed. After your first treatment you may find that you need more or less help than anticipated. You may be fine with driving yourself to and from your treatments. You may find that you need more housekeeping help or child care hours than you thought.

√ **Start a journal.** Some people find that keeping a journal or a diary is a helpful way to keep track of how they feel, the things they learned, and helpful books and websites. Some people find that when they record their feelings, they don't have to carry all their concerns in their minds. It also helps them gain insight and lower their stress. Some people "journal" through writing letters or e-mails as they share their experiences with close friends. Save a copy of those letters for yourself. That becomes your journal—a document of your experiences during this time.

Get Ready

There are many things you can do before your treatment that will help things go more smoothly afterward. Here are some suggestions:

√ **See your dentist.** If possible, see your dentist to get your teeth cleaned and any necessary dental work done before you start chemo. Many chemotherapy medicines lower your ability to fight infection and your blood's ability to clot. Although dental emergencies can occur at any time, it's best to avoid invasive procedures that increase your risk of infection or bleeding while you're in treatment.

√ **Stock up.** Go shopping for the foods, juices, and supplies that you'll want to have available for the first few days after your treatment. You'll be told to "push fluids" and eat bland foods that are easily digested. So stock up on drinks (juices, sports drinks, Popsicles, watermelon, soup, broth, and herbal tea) and foods (potatoes, rice, cereal, pasta, cheese and crackers). Chapter 7 ("Maintaining Good Nutrition") has more suggestions. Also pick up a thermometer, a soft toothbrush, baking soda, disposable hand wipes, and sunscreen. After your first treatment, you'll have a better idea of the kinds of foods, fluids, and supplies you want to have on hand.

√ **Confirm arrangements.** It's a good idea to have someone drive you or accompany you on public transportation to your first chemo treatment. Some of the medications you receive may make you too sleepy to drive or travel alone. After your first treatment, you'll be able to better predict how you'll feel and what your transportation needs will be. Confirm your schedule with the people helping you at work and at home.

√ **Buy head coverings.** If hair loss (or hair thinning) is one of the side effects of your chemotherapy treatment, plan ahead. Many people cut their hair to a shorter style before the first treatment. If you plan to buy a wig, consider making your selection before you lose all your hair so that you can more accurately match your usual hair color and style. Even if you plan to wear a wig some of the time, be sure to stock up on other head coverings. There'll be times when you'll want to wear just a hat or scarf. Chapter 9 ("Coping with Hair Loss and Skin Changes") has more information.

√ **Take classes.** Get information about support groups or classes available in your area. The American Cancer Society sponsors a class called "Look Good, Feel Better" presented by cosmetologists who teach women creative ideas about how to use makeup, hats, scarves, and wigs during treatment. If you had surgery for cancer that affected your lymph nodes, you want to avoid *lymphedema*, a condition that can cause painful swelling. There may be classes taught by a lymphedema specialist who can teach you about the prevention and treatment of this problem. Also, you can attend a class taught by a nutritionist who specializes in oncology to learn more about how to maintain good nutrition before, during, and after chemotherapy.

√ **Plan an activity to do during your treatment.** Some treatments require that you spend many hours in the clinic. You may want to doze or watch TV for a while or bring some other activity to help the time pass. Bring a book or magazine, do word puzzles, listen to music, watch a DVD, or knit. If a friend comes with you, you might enjoy playing cards, Scrabble, or other games.

√ **Fill your prescriptions.** Your doctor may want you to take medicine at home. For instance, you may need medication to prevent or relieve nausea. You may need a laxative or a medication to prevent or relieve diarrhea. Or you may need an antibiotic. Ask your doctor to give you the prescriptions before your day of treatment so that you can have them filled ahead of time. Then bring the medications with you to the clinic so that your nurse can review the instructions before you go home. Sometimes there's a delay in filling the prescriptions. Some medications require prior authorization, and that can take some time. If your insurance company won't authorize a medication, your doctor may be able to substitute a different one that will be as effective but less expensive.

√ **Get your house ready.** Get basic housework done before your treatment, because you may feel too tired to do it later. Get the laundry done. Clean your home thoroughly to reduce the risk of infection. Shop, cook, and freeze meals for later. You'll feel better if your home environment is clean and organized, and has the food and supplies you'll need.

√ **The night before chemo.** Unless you've been instructed otherwise, there's no reason to fast or have an empty stomach before your treatment. You'll be given medications to prevent nausea, so you'll be able to eat and drink during your treatment. Still, it's a good idea to avoid fried foods or anything that may upset your stomach. Eat a bland dinner the night before chemo and plan to eat a bland, light breakfast in the morning. Try to get a good night's sleep.

DURING YOUR CHEMO TREATMENT

Here are some suggestions to help make the day of your treatment go more smoothly.

√ **Dress comfortably.** Loose, layered clothing is a good idea so that you can stay comfortable whatever the room temperature. Wear a shirt with sleeves that can easily be rolled up for the nurse to start your IV in your arm and take your blood pressure. Wear a shirt with an open neck if you have a chest port so that the nurse can easily access it for your IV.

√ **Bring whatever you may need for the hours you'll be at the clinic.** Here are some suggestions:

- Activities (books, music, games)

- Food, snacks, drinks

- Your chemo binder (to keep copies of your labs, scheduled appointments, and so on)

- Your list of questions for your doctor or nurse

- Your regular medicines, such as pain meds or diabetes meds, to take if their scheduled times coincide with your treatment appointment

- Your filled prescription of antinausea meds or other meds you'll need to take after chemotherapy (review them with your nurse so that you're sure how and when to take them)

- Important phone numbers for contacting your family or friends in case you need to reach them

- The phone number of your local pharmacy

- A list of your allergies

√ **Stay connected.** Ask your nurse to explain things so that you understand what's happening. If you notice any unusual feeling, such as pain, sweating, itching, or nausea, tell your nurses right away. Also let them know other things that would add to your comfort. You may want the lights dimmed, the TV channel changed, a warm blanket, more juice, or help getting to the toilet. If you're at the clinic for a number of hours (and aren't too sleepy), you may be able to consult with the social worker or nutritionist while you're there.

AFTER YOUR CHEMO TREATMENT

Once you get home, there are many things you can do to feel comfortable and prevent or manage the possible side effects of treatment.

√ **Stay hydrated.** Drink eight to ten (eight-ounce) glasses of fluids daily. This should include a variety of fluids. Juices, sports drinks, soup, broth, herbal tea, watermelon, and Popsicles are good choices. This will help your body eliminate the chemotherapy and help you to feel better. Chapter 7 ("Maintaining Good Nutrition") has more fluid suggestions.

√ **Take your medicines as directed.** If your doctor or nurse recommends taking medicine to prevent a problem (nausea, constipation, diarrhea, and so on), follow these instructions exactly to avoid these unpleasant side effects. If you're unable to take the medicines for any reason, call the clinic or the on-call physician to advise you about what to do. Medicines to relieve side effects are more effective if you take them as soon as you experience the problem rather than wait until you're very uncomfortable. Chapter 5 ("Preventing Nausea") and Chapter 6 ("Coping with Other Digestion Changes") have more suggestions.

√ **Keep a record of any side effects you experience.** Note when it occurred, what made it better, and what made it worse. Also, keep track of the medicine you took to relieve the problem, when you took it, and how effective it was. This will help your doctor decide if there should be a change in the medicine or dosage for more effective relief.

√ **Monitor your temperature.** Your doctor or nurse may instruct you to take your temperature twice a day for a period of time. But if you're feeling ill in any way (headache, cold, cough, achiness, chills), take your temperature (before brushing your teeth, eating, or drinking) and call the clinic, even if you don't have a fever. Be sure to call your doctor or nurse if your temperature ever goes above 100.5°F (not 105.0°F or 38°C). This could be an early sign of infection.

√ **Reduce your risk of infection.** You may be more susceptible to infection during this time, so do everything you can to lower your chances of exposure. Wash your hands frequently and thoroughly with soap and water. Have your family members wash their hands often, too, especially if they're preparing food. Try to stay away from people who are sick, and avoid crowded, enclosed spaces where you would be exposed to people who may cough or sneeze near you. Chapter 3 ("Understanding Blood Tests") has more suggestions.

√ **Keep your mouth clean and healthy.** Use frequent, gentle mouth care. Brush with a soft toothbrush and rinse with a solution of one teaspoon of baking soda in one cup of warm water. This will get rid of any acidy taste and promote healing of your mucous membranes. Let your doctor know if your mouth is painful, if you have any white, patchy areas, or if any sores develop. There are medications that can provide relief and healing.

√ **Avoid alcohol, spicy foods, and acidic foods and juices.** They can irritate your stomach lining and cause or worsen nausea, heartburn, or abdominal pain.

√ **Get plenty of rest.** Fatigue is the most common side effect of all cancer treatments, so listen to your body. It's working hard to rid you of the waste products of chemo and to repair normal cells. If you're tired, sit down, put your feet up, and close your eyes for a while. Try to alternate rest periods with active periods. Chapter 8 ("Coping with Fatigue") has more suggestions.

√ **Stay active.** If you can, keep active and continue to exercise. Even on the days when you feel tired or wiped out, be sure to take a walk around your house or outdoors. Being active helps relieve nausea, improves your appetite, helps you sleep better at night, and lifts your spirits. It also helps your breathing and lessens the chance of developing blood clots in your legs.

√ **Report any problems.** Call your doctor or nurse with any problems—even if you think they may not be significant. Call if you can't control nausea or if you're vomiting. Call if you have diarrhea or constipation or if you feel yourself getting dehydrated because you haven't been able to drink sufficient fluids. Call if your mouth is sore or if you're having trouble swallowing. Call if you're having any bleeding or pain. Also, report any sign of infection, such as fever, chills, sore throat, productive cough, difficulty urinating, or a skin cut that's swollen or red. Don't wait until your next appointment, which may be a week or more away. Since your infection-fighting capacity is compromised by the chemo, you may need an antibiotic to fight the infection. Let your doctor assess the problem (big or small) and resolve it quickly.

√ **Protect others.** You'll be excreting the chemotherapy in your body fluids and waste products, such as urine and stool. So it's recommended that for forty-eight hours after each chemotherapy treatment, you flush the toilet twice each time you use it. If you're sexually active, be sure to use a condom during sex for a few days after each treatment. This will protect your partner from any chemo that may be in your semen or vaginal fluid.

√ **Keep your appointments.** Your doctor will probably order lab tests and a return visit about a week after your treatment to check your blood counts and to see how you're doing. It's important to keep these appointments so that any problems can be detected early. Treating a potential problem early is much more effective than waiting until the problem becomes severe. Take your notebook with you to these visits to get your questions and concerns addressed.

IN CONCLUSION

The best way to prepare for the start of chemo is to get the information you need so that you know how to plan and organize. Part of the stress of facing treatment is that you're dealing with the unknown. You're not sure how you'll feel during and after your treatment or when you get home. After your first treatment, you'll likely feel much less anxious. You'll develop your own coping strategies and a checklist of things to remember. You'll have more confidence knowing what you can do to prevent problems and how and when to get help if problems arise. You'll be able to trust your doctor and nurses and your friends and family to help you get through this challenging time.

Chapter 16

Life After Cancer Treatments: Being a Survivor

When we began this book, we said that when you're facing cancer treatments for the first time, it can feel as if you've been dropped off behind enemy lines during a war. You don't know the language or the terrain, and you don't know what's expected. But you got through it. You learned the language and medical terminology; mobilized your energy and resolve; and rearranged your life, your job, and your family. You've educated yourself, reached out for help, made decisions, endured, and prevailed through it all. Now that your treatment is completed, you may feel like a soldier coming back after a long and difficult battle. You're relieved and grateful to be home and back to "normal life," but you may feel a little disoriented for a while. You may have many questions about what you can expect during this time of transition. You may have some emotions that surprise you, and some may seem contradictory. You may feel grateful and angry. You may feel full of life and hope at times, yet at other times depressed or fearful. Your relationships with others, even your place in the world, may feel unsettled.

Everyone has a unique journey through treatment and the period after treatment. No one can tell you what you'll feel or exactly what you can do to get through this transition. It will depend on many things, such as the kind of cancer you had, the goals of treatment, and the kind of chemotherapy you received. It will depend on the impact it had on your life, your family, and your finances. It will depend on the long-term physical changes or limitations you're dealing with. It will depend on your age, personality, coping style, and so on.

Getting back to normal both physically and psychologically may take some time. As you regain your physical strength and resume your previous roles and activities, you'll feel more comfortable being "home" again. This chapter is a different kind of survival guide. It discusses some of the issues and challenges many people face after cancer treatments and offer some suggestions about what you can do to help yourself along the way.

PHYSICAL CHANGES

Just because you're no longer receiving treatment doesn't mean that you're not under the care and supervision of your oncologist. You may not be at the clinic as often, but your doctor will continue to follow you as your immune system recovers, your energy returns, and the residual side effects of treatment fade. Your oncologist is still a very important resource for you even after your chemotherapy treatments are over. He or she will continue to follow your blood tests, which show how your white cells, platelets, and red cells are recovering. A physical exam, lab tests, and other diagnostic tests can evaluate your heart and lungs, kidney, liver, thyroid, and hormone levels.

Side Effects After Treatment

Problems such as nausea, queasiness, loss of appetite, and taste changes that are associated with your chemotherapy will fade over the first month after treatment. You'll find that food—planning meals, cooking, or just eating—will be more interesting to you. You'll also find that fatigue slowly decreases as well. You may not be aware of the improvement day by day, but if you look back to how you felt a week ago, you'll see the change. If the chemotherapy caused hair loss or thinning, you'll start to notice it growing back. It may be several months before you feel comfortable going without a head covering if you wear a wig, hat, or scarf, but it's exciting to see the change. You'll find that your skin is less dry and your nails are less fragile. These side effects are directly caused by chemotherapy's effect on frequently dividing cells, and without chemotherapy, those parts of your body return to normal.

Chemotherapy can also cause side effects that can persist for a time, but many of those will eventually resolve. It may take a while for your bone marrow (the blood-cell factory) to recover. Even after your treatment is completed, you may find that your red cells (which carry oxygen), white cells (which fight infection), or platelets (which help your blood clot) remain slightly below normal. Therefore you should still let your oncologist know before you plan to have dental work or any other invasive procedure. Your oncologist will tell you when it's safe to proceed and what precautions you need to take.

Some side effects from cancer treatments can persist longer—or even be permanent. For instance, some chemotherapy medicines can cause damage to the nerves of your fingers or feet and toes. You may experience numbness, tingling, or even pain. As described in chapter 10, this is called peripheral neuropathy. There are some medications that can help with this problem, and many people find that neuropathy improves over time, but it may take many months.

Some people experience physical changes caused by cancer, surgery, or other cancer-fighting treatments that will always be with them. Scars, the loss of a body part (whether visible or not), a colostomy after colon or rectal surgery, lymphedema after breast surgery, and infertility are examples of the challenges some people face at the end of their treatments.

Things That Can Help

Keep track of the physical symptoms you're having and whether or not they seem to be getting better or worse over time. Many symptoms will fade out over the weeks and months following chemo. But if they don't, your doctor may have some suggestions or can refer you to another specialist who can help. You might benefit from the services of a physical therapist to regain strength, balance, or flexibility. You may benefit from the lymphedema clinic if you develop swelling in your arms or legs. A pain-management specialist can help you deal with nerve pain or other pains that persist. An ophthalmologist can treat eye problems, such as dryness or excessive tearing. There are medications that can help with hot flashes, vaginal dryness, or loss of sexual libido, which can result from changes in hormone levels after treatment.

You may be facing further surgery for reconstruction or for reversing the effects of a previous surgery (reversing a colostomy, for example, or breast reconstruction). If you really have a choice about when to proceed with further procedures, do what feels right for you. Some people want to get all the medical procedures over with as soon as possible. Other people want to take their time to regain their strength and energy before undergoing any more physical stress. They'll explore possible treatments, assess the options, and make those decisions later. Ask your oncologist what's recommended and why.

Take steps to promote your long-term health and well-being. Diet and exercise is a frequently discussed subject. A healthy diet with lots of fresh fruits and vegetables, lean meat (or other protein sources), and whole grains is highly recommended, as well as avoiding sugar, "bad" fats, and empty calories. This advice is the basis for every healthy diet. Being physically active within our physical capability is also something that we all should do. Now that your treatment is over and you're regaining your strength and appetite, it's a good time to reconsider how to integrate these healthy changes into your life for your future health and well-being.

Diet. Resist the impulse to make huge changes all at once in your diet. This is not the time to suddenly decide to be a vegan or to eat a strict macrobiotic diet unless this is something you've done and enjoyed in the past. As your appetite and sense of taste improve, you can consider food again without worrying about nausea or queasiness, diarrhea, constipation, and other digestion problems that you may have dealt with during treatment. Of course, there are many reasons why some people still have some problems with eating, digestion, or elimination that persist after treatment. But eating a healthy, balanced diet that's familiar and enjoyable is a good place to start. The nutritionist at your clinic will be able to help you make a plan. There are also many books, articles, cookbooks, and recipes in bookstores and online that can give you good ideas about how to shop and prepare food in a healthy way to support a healthy body.

Exercise. If fatigue or nausea limited your activities during treatment, you'll be glad when they're no longer a problem. The exercise you choose depends, of course, on your physical limitations, interests, and available time. Just taking a walk each day is a good place to start. The fresh air, the sights and sounds of the environment, breathing deeply, and feeling your body moving in space are all things that contribute to your well-being. No matter what activity you choose, start slowly and increase the time and distance gradually. Stop when you're tired and proceed when you're able. You'll feel encouraged when you realize that you can go farther with less fatigue. As with any exercise program, you have to set time aside each day to do it. That's why simpler and more accessible activities are easier to keep up. Having a friend come along also helps you stick with the program. The goal is to create a routine that you're likely to stick to; it need not entail a huge commitment of time, expensive equipment, or membership in a health club. Once you regain your strength, you can explore or resume other activities, such as biking, hiking, swimming, and tennis, that are fun and get you out and moving.

Primary care. Reconnect with your primary-care doctor. During your cancer treatments, your oncologist probably managed most of your medical care. Your oncologist may have consulted with your primary-care doctor or sent you to other specialists if necessary. But since any and all preexisting medical problems had to be considered in light of your treatments, you probably consulted with the oncology clinic first. Once your active treatment is complete, your oncologist will continue to follow you closely for several more months as your immune system recovers and any side effects of treatment slowly resolve.

But eventually you should reestablish your relationship with your primary doctor or other specialists you consulted before. For example, you may have seen a cardiologist for management of high blood pressure or an endocrinologist for management of diabetes. You'll also need a doctor for routine screenings (lab tests, mammograms, Pap smears, prostate exams, colonoscopy), immunizations, and cholesterol management, as well as to renew routine prescriptions or to treat a cold or virus.

It's a good idea to have a copy of your treatment records and lab reports sent to your primary physician and specialists. That way everyone knows what medications you're taking (or have stopped taking) during chemotherapy, what side effects from treatment you may still be experiencing, or any other changes that affect your health.

EMOTIONAL ISSUES

Just to get through cancer treatments took an enormous amount of determination, focus, and courage. There may have been little time to adjust or prepare. You had to educate yourself and make treatment decisions before you felt confident. You were required to meet and trust a team of medical professionals whom you hardly knew. You had to rearrange your family, your work, your finances, and your priorities. Clinic appointments filled your weeks, and just eating, drinking, digesting, and sleeping were the "activities" that filled each day. Of course, you had many fears, but there wasn't a lot of time to process or resolve much of it. It was war.

Anxiety

Although you looked forward to the end of the treatment phase and to resuming your regular life, it's common to experience some anxiety after treatment ends. Some people say that as long as they were in treatment, they were "fighting" cancer. Now, without treatment, they feel anxious that they're no longer actively engaged in the fight. Although you're probably glad to spend less time at the clinic, the clinic has probably been a source of advice and support. Some people miss not having the nurses or their doctors as available as they had been.

Post-Traumatic Stress

As you look back to the early days of your diagnosis, you can see that just being told that you had cancer was in itself traumatic. The following months of treatment were a challenge to your body and soul. After any traumatic event, there are lots of emotions and adjustments that you may not have had a chance to work through. It's like running a marathon. You have to be focused on the finish line, sustaining yourself as best you can through the grueling ordeal. Once the race is over, you start to experience the inevitable sore muscles, blistered feet, and total exhaustion.

After cancer treatments, it's normal to need time and support to process the experience. You may not feel like your old self, because the struggle itself may have changed your sense of self. You may feel pride that you were able to rise to the occasion, and grateful to have gotten through it. Many people say that they found resources within themselves that they never knew they had. Yet you may be left with other feelings (fear, anger, depression, grief) that you couldn't afford to experience while going through treatment. Even the term "cancer survivor" implies strength and courage but also the seriousness of the threat that was overcome. It will take time and the support of your family and friends for you to integrate what you've been through into a new sense of self.

Fears About Recurrence

At the end of treatment you want your doctor to assure you that the cancer is gone forever—that you don't ever have to worry about cancer again. But even if your cancer is very unlikely to recur, you're not given a 100 percent guarantee. So you have to live with a degree of uncertainty, when what you really want is certainty. Fears about recurrence may ebb and flow. They may be worse around the time of your checkup visits or after a scan or lab test. They may be triggered by any new physical discomfort, change, ache, or pain. Reading an article or seeing a show on TV may trigger fears.

Things That Can Help

Your feelings are complex and unique. If you talk to other people who are in this post-treatment transition, you'll hear a wide range of issues and many different ways that people find the paths of their own emotional healing.

The good news is that most people find that periods of anxiety lessen over time, the further they are from treatment. Even though there are still triggers that can set you back, over time they're fewer and you'll be more experienced in managing them. Here are some suggestions about what you can do to feel better when your emotions seem overwhelming. The techniques described in chapter 14 ("Relaxation and Stress Reduction") can be helpful as well.

Try to stay in the present. When you feel fearful, you're probably focusing on the future—events that haven't happened and outcomes you can neither know nor control. But when you're in the grip of anxiety, it's tempting to project yourself into a frightful future to prepare for potential problems that may not even occur. You experience the worry again and again, which makes your anxiety worse.

Many people find that if they return to the present, they can lessen their anxiety. You can do that by focusing on all the sensations, sounds, and colors of your immediate environment. A good way to start is to just pay attention to your breath. You don't have to breathe any special way; just notice the flow of air and the rise and fall of your chest. Then notice the sights and sounds of your immediate environment. Look at the shape, color, and texture of the objects around you as if you're planning to draw or paint the scene. Then pay attention to the pressure of the floor on the soles of your feet, the pressure of the chair in which you sit, the feel of your clothes on your body, and so on. When you're aware that your mind wanders to future worries, just refocus on the present moment again until the anxiety subsides.

Learn what's calming to you. Is there an activity you enjoy that helps you feel focused and calm? Gardening, listening to music, practicing the piano, working with wood or other crafts, taking a walk with a friend, praying, and watching a movie are some suggestions.

Think of the activity that will work for you. Is there a comforting word or phrase that you can repeat to yourself aloud or in your mind? Consider words such as "peace," "calmness," "love," "quiet," "Jesus" or phrases such as "I can get through this," "_____ is here for me," "I can't know the future," and "I have come so far."

Is there a pleasant ritual that you find relaxing? Sitting down with a cup of tea, walking the dog, doing the daily crossword puzzle, taking a shower, and getting a foot massage are activities that help some people feel more calm.

Is there an object or a piece of clothing or jewelry that can function as a "good-luck charm"? It can be something you can take with you, wear, or put in your pocket. When you see or touch it, you can feel comforted by remembering its significance.

Is there a friend or family member who always seems to make you feel better? That's the person to bring with you when you go for a scan or doctor's visit that causes anxiety. It could be someone who'll provide distraction or just a calm presence.

Is there some special reward you can give yourself after getting through a difficult event? It may help to plan something such as having lunch with a friend or buying tickets to a concert or movie so that you have something to look forward to.

Once you realize that you can successfully lower your anxiety, you'll feel more in control. Inevitably there will still be anxiety-triggering circumstances. But anxiety doesn't have to be overwhelming. You can find comfort and support within yourself by focusing on thoughts and activities that are calming.

GETTING BACK TO NORMAL

Be patient with yourself. It will take a while to regain your energy. Recovery is not a straight road. There may be days when you feel stronger, both physically and emotionally, and other days when you may feel tired and overwhelmed. So take it slowly and don't try to tackle everything all at once. You may still need someone to help with child care or household chores for a while. You may need to return to work on a part-time basis (working fewer hours per day or fewer days per week) until you see how you feel.

Be patient with others. They may not know what it is that you need from them, especially if what you need changes each day. Some days you may feel tired and need rest. Other days you may be full of energy. Some days you need someone to talk to about your treatment experiences. Other days you want to put those experiences far behind you. When you let people know what your needs are, they're more likely to meet them. Let people know that you may need to cancel a social event if you find that you're too tired that day. Or you can tell your friends that you want the afternoon to be a "no cancer zone," in which conversations about cancer aren't welcome.

Telling your story. There are times when you may need to talk about what you went through: your fears and struggles during treatment as well as how you feel during this transition. Some friends or family members may not understand that you may need to process what you've been through. They might feel that you shouldn't dwell on past events and that you should be optimistic about the future. Or there may be others who just cannot hear your story, because they're overwhelmed with their own fears about cancer or cancer treatments. Think carefully about who in your life is able to really listen, and let those people know what you need from them (whether it's time, patience, understanding, respect for your privacy, or an accepting quiet witness to your story). Tell them what you don't need from them (for instance, advice, problem solving, cheering up, pity). You may need to tell the story a number of times as you integrate what you've been through with who you are now.

Writing your story. Keeping a journal of your feelings during this time is a good way to acknowledge all your emotions. In the book *Picking Up the Pieces* (2006), authors Sherrie Magee and Kathy Scalzo recommend taking time at the end of each day to sit quietly with your thoughts and write short answers to these questions:

- What's happening to my body?

- How am I feeling emotionally?

- When I let my thoughts wander, what do I find myself thinking about?

- Whom did I connect with today?

- What gave me a sense of peace? (67)

This becomes a "change-tracking system, progress map, and diary all in one" (69). Some people join a writing group or a poetry group to have a place to express their feelings creatively. You can tell your story through any artistic expression, such as painting, dancing, quilting, or music.

Reaching out for help. You're not alone. There are many, many people who have faced some of the same challenges that you're dealing with. Many cancer clinics have support groups for people who have completed treatment. You'll find validation by listening to others who are going through this transition, even if the kind of cancer they had or their prognosis differs from your own. They know how you're feeling. People find strength, both physically and emotionally, in different ways. You can also help others if and when you share your story, your strategies, and your successes.

Sometimes feelings can be really debilitating. If you're constantly overwhelmed with anxiety and panic or if depression has you immobilized, you can't do the things that will help you feel better. You may benefit from some counseling with a professional who is experienced in helping people deal with anxiety and depression associated with health problems. Your clinic may have a counselor on staff, or your doctor may be able to refer you to someone who can evaluate what kind of assistance you need. Sometimes just being able to talk to someone outside of your family can be a real help. If necessary, you can be referred to a physician who can evaluate your need for medications to help you get through this time. Chapter 13 ("Mind and Body"), written by Dr. Burton Presberg, has more helpful information.

IN CONCLUSION

This period after your treatment ends is a time of transition. You've been through a battle and survived it. You may feel disoriented at first, and normal life may feel like unfamiliar territory for a while. But in time you'll find your way back to a new "normal," with all its inherent joys and problems. Some people are relieved to resume their jobs and their roles in their families and communities. Some want to make changes so that they have a job with less stress or more meaning. Some want to change their priorities so that they can spend more time with their families, pursue new hobbies or interests, or develop an underexplored talent. For some it's a time for spiritual growth and reaffirmation of their faith. Transitions are often uncomfortable at first. You know that from all the other transitions you've experienced in your life. But through all the changes, your basic sense of self remains. Your values and purpose give you your direction. Your inner strengths and resilience will sustain you.

Judith McKay, RN, OCN, received her degree from California State University, Hayward, and has been an oncology nurse involved in patient education for more than twenty-five years. She helped develop and taught chemotherapy orientation classes at the Alta Bates Summit Comprehensive Cancer Center in Berkeley, CA, where she currently works. McKay is coauthor of *When Anger Hurts* and contributed to the best-seller *Self-Esteem*.

Tamera Schacher, RN, OCN, MSN, is an oncology-certified nurse and a board-certified family nurse practitioner. She trained to become a registered nurse at the University of Nevada, Las Vegas, and received her master of science in nursing and family nurse practitioner degrees at Sonoma State University. For the past five years, she has worked at the Alta Bates Summit Comprehensive Cancer Center.

Index

nutritional supplements for, 109-110; sample menu for, 108

chemoreceptor trigger zone (CTZ), 69

chemotherapy, 2, 14-18; blood cells and, 17, 33, 38; combinations of drugs for, 16; coping with stress of, 54-56; how it works, 14-15; managing effects following, 239-241; medical treatments during, 47; nutrition and, 105-115, 235-236; preparing for, 231-239; protecting others from, 241; recovery process after, 243-254; side effects of, 17-18, 87-88, 139, 244-245; staying comfortable during, 53-54; targeted therapies and, 15-16

chest ports, 61-62

Chew, Tinrin, 4, 103, 123

chi, 158, 209

chronic stress, 216

cisplatin, 155, 161

clinical trials, 27-28

clotting factors, 45

clove tea, 121

cochlea, 161

cognitive impairment, 163-170

cold sensitivity, 155-156

colon, 88

colony-stimulating factor (CSF), 40

community resources, 135

Compazine, 73, 75, 76, 89

complementary therapies, 209-210

complete blood count (CBC), 32, 34

computed tomography (CT) scans, 21

concentration problems, 163-170

constipation, 72, 99-101; medications to relieve, 100-101; nutritional recommendations for,

119; peripheral neuropathy and, 160-161; prevention of, 99-100, 160-161

coping with cancer, 206-210; complementary therapies for, 209-210; counseling/therapy for, 206-207; individual styles of, 211; religion/spirituality for, 208-209; support groups for, 207-208; supportive thoughts for, 84-85

counseling, 206-207

cuffs, 66

cultures, 41-42

D

Decadron, 73, 76, 130

deep breathing, 217-218

dehydration, 78-80; constipation and, 99; dealing with, 79-80; diarrhea and, 98; dry mouth and, 89; signs of, 78; WHO solution for, 121

delayed nausea, 76

dental work, 235, 245

dentures, 91

depression, 166, 201-202

dexamethasone, 73, 76, 130

diagnosis, 12-13

diarrhea, 97-99; caused by infections, 97, 98-99; nutritional recommendations for, 120-122; reasons for developing, 97; suggestions for dealing with, 98

diet: appetite problems and, 94-95, 122; chemo cycles and, 105-115; constipation and, 99-100, 119; diarrhea and, 98, 120-122; dry mouth and, 89; fatigue and, 136-137; heartburn and, 96; menu samples for, 108, 115; post-treatment, 246-247; taste changes

and, 92-93, 117-118. *See also*
foods; nutrition
Diflucan, 93
digestion problems, 17, 87-101;
appetite problems, 94-95;
chemotherapy and, 87-88, 97;
constipation, 99-101; diarrhea,
97-99; food aversions, 95;
heartburn, 95-97; mouth/throat
problems, 89-93; nutritional
recommendations for, 116-122;
taste changes, 92-93, 94; yeast
infections, 93
digestive system, 88
diphenhydramine, 74, 89
disability options, 233
DNA, 7, 10
docetaxel, 155, 157
docosahexaenoic acid (DHA), 114
dolasetron, 71
donor eggs/embryos, 195
donor sperm, 194
dopamine, 73
Doxil, 148
dronabinol, 74
drugs: antibiotic, 41, 42;
anticonvulsant, 157;
antidepressant, 157, 202; anti-
EGFR, 148; antinausea, 70-74,
75-76, 77, 82; brain function
and, 165; chemotherapy, 14-17;
combinations of, 16; constipation,
100-101; diarrhea, 99; heartburn,
96-97; peripheral neuropathy,
157-158; targeted therapy, 15-16
dry mouth, 89
dry skin, 145-146
dysplasia, 11

E

eating habits. *See* diet; nutrition

edema, 45
eggs (ova), 185-186; donor embryos
and, 195; fertilization of, 186,
187-188; freezing of, 191
eicosapentaenoic acid (EPA), 114
ejaculation, 185
electrolytes, 44
Eloxatin, 155
embryo freezing, 190-191
Emend, 72
emetic potential, 70
emotions, 200-203; post-treatment,
248-251; sadness vs. depression,
201-202; social support and,
202-203
endorphins, 166
enemas, 101
energy conservation, 133-135
enzymes, 45
eosinophils, 37
epidermal growth factor receptors
(EGFRs), 148
Erbitux, 148
erlotinib, 148
erythrocytes, 34
erythropoietin, 36, 131
esophagitis, 90
esophagus, 88
estrogen, 173, 176
exercise: brain function and, 167;
fatigue and, 132-133; post-
treatment, 247; sleep and, 135.
See also physical activity

F

Family Medical Leave Act (FMLA),
233
fatigue, 94, 125-138; brain function
and, 164-165; cancer as cause of,
126; chemotherapy and, 125, 127,
129-130; energy conservation

and, 133-135; exercise and, 132-133; getting medical help for, 130-131; infection/fever and, 128; low blood counts and, 127-128; nutrition and, 136-137; pain as cause of, 129; sleep and, 135-136; social support and, 137-138; stress/anxiety and, 129; suggestions for dealing with, 132-138; treatments for cancer and, 126-127

fats, 112

Fertile Hope, 197

fertility, 183-197; basics of, 184-186; evaluating after treatment, 193; getting medical information about, 183-184; and infertility treatment costs, 196-197; men's issues and options with, 186-189, 194; women's issues and options with, 189-193, 195-196

fertilization, 186

fever, 128, 131

fiber supplements, 101

fight-or-flight response, 215

5HT3 antagonists, 71, 76

fluconazole, 93

fluids: chemo phase guidelines for, 105-107; constipation and, 99; consumption of, 79, 83; dehydration and, 78-80; diarrhea and loss of, 98; dry mouth and, 89; importance of, 77-78, 83; mouth soreness and, 91; rebuilding phase guidelines for, 110

flushed skin, 147

foods: aversions to, 95; chemo phase guidelines for, 107-108; high-fiber, 99-100; hot or spicy, 91; rebuilding phase guidelines

for, 111-112; taste changes and, 92-93, 117-118. *See also* diet; nutrition

foreign cells, 10

fruits, 111

furosemide, 89

G

gastric reflux, 96

gastrointestinal (GI) tract, 17

G-CSF, 40

gefitinib, 148

Get Out of Your Mind and Into Your Life (Hayes and Smith), 223

glutamine, 114, 157

grains, 112

granisetron, 71, 99

granulocytes, 36, 40

gynecologists, 175

H

H2 blockers, 96

hair loss, 17, 139-145; coping with, 141-144; progress of, 140-141; reasons for, 140; regrowth of hair following, 145; thinning hair and, 144

hand-foot syndrome, 148-149

hats, 143

head wraps, 143

headaches, 72

health care professionals: communicating with, 47; primary-care doctors, 247-248

hearing loss, 161-162

heartburn, 95-97; explanation of, 95-96; medications for relieving, 96-97

hematocrit (Hct) measurement, 35

hemoglobin (Hgb) test, 34-35

Hexadrol, 73

high-fiber foods, 99-100
histamine, 95
hormone changes, 173-174
hormone replacement therapy
    (HRT), 174
hormone-blocking medicines, 15
housework, 237
humor, 211
hydrochloric acid, 95
hyperplasia, 11

I
ibuprofen, 157
imagery: breathing and, 218; retreat
    scripts using, 219-220
immune system: cells protected by,
    9; infections and, 41
Imodium, 99
implanted vascular access devices,
    61-64; arm ports, 63; chest ports,
    61-62
in vitro fertilization (IVF), 187-188
infections, 40-42; antibiotics for
    fighting, 41, 42, 131; cultures
    for determining, 41-42; diarrhea
    caused by, 97, 98-99;fatigue
    caused by, 128; reducing risk of,
    240; VADs and, 66-67; yeast, 93
infertility issues. See fertility
insurance coverage: importance
    of understanding, 232; second
    opinions and, 26
interferons, 16, 127
interleukin-2, 127
intracytoplasmic sperm injection
    (ICSI), 188
intramuscular (IM) injections, 44
intrauterine insemination (IUI), 188
invasive cells, 11
Iressa, 148
iron supplements, 131

IV catheters, 51, 58-68; implanted
    ports for, 61-64; peripherally
    inserted central, 59-60; potential
    problems with, 66-68; tunneled,
    64-66
IV treatments, 49-68; bags/bottles/
    tubes for, 52-53; continuous, 53;
    handling problems with, 56-57;
    pain caused by, 57; pumps for,
    52, 53; starting, 51-52; veins used
    for, 50-51; venous access devices
    for, 58-68

J
Jacobson, Edmund, 223
journal writing, 235, 252-253

K
Kegel exercises, 176
Kytril, 71, 99

L
lab tests, 21; cultures as, 41-42;
    reviewing results of, 45-46. See
    also blood tests
Lasix, 89
laughter, 211
laxatives, 100-101
Leave Your Mind Behind: The
    Everyday Practice of Finding
    Stillness Amid Rushing Thoughts
    (McKay and Sutker), 223
leukocytes, 36
lidocaine, 64
lip balms, 91
liposomal doxorubicin, 148
local anesthetics, 64
Lomotil, 99
"Look Good, Feel Better" program,
    152, 236
loperamide, 99

throat problems. *See* mouth/throat problems

thrush, 93

time management, 133-135

tingling sensations, 154, 155

tinnitus, 162

topical anesthetic, 92

tourniquets, 50

treatment conference, 22

treatment plans, 19-30; changes made to, 29; clinical trials and, 27-28; determining effectiveness of, 28-29; foundations of, 19-22; getting a second opinion about, 26; making use of consultations about, 24-25; preparing to begin, 232; questions to ask about, 22-23, 24

treatments, 2-3, 13-16; chemotherapy, 14-15; radiation, 14; recovery after, 243-254; surgery, 13; targeted therapies, 15-16

tumor board, 22

tumor markers, 21, 46-47

tunneled catheters, 64-66

U

ultrasound, 21, 59

urologists, 175

V

vaccines, 10

vegetables, 111

veins, 49-51, 58

Velban, 160

venous access devices (VADs), 58-68; implanted, 61-64; peripherally inserted central catheters, 59-60; potential problems with, 66-68; tunneled catheters, 64-66

vinblastine, 160

vinca alkaloids, 160

vincristine, 99, 160

visualization, 219-220

vitamins, 109-110, 113

vomiting: anticipatory nausea and, 77; chemotherapy and, 70. *See also* nausea

W

watermelon, 106-107

weight gain/loss, 104

white blood cells, 9, 36-40; chemotherapy and, 38; dealing with drop in, 39-40; stimulating production of, 40; types of, 36-38

wigs, 141-144; alternatives to, 143-144; considerations for buying, 142-143

women: fertility issues for, 189-193; sexuality help for, 176

work options, 233

World Health Organization (WHO), 121

writing your story, 252-253

X

Xeloda, 148

X-rays, 21

Y

yeast infections, 93

Z

Zofran, 71, 99

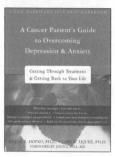
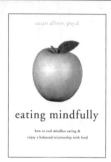
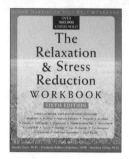
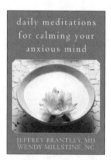
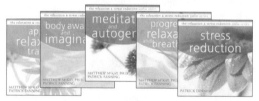
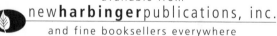